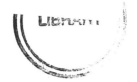
THE
PARAS
ULTIMATE
FITNESS

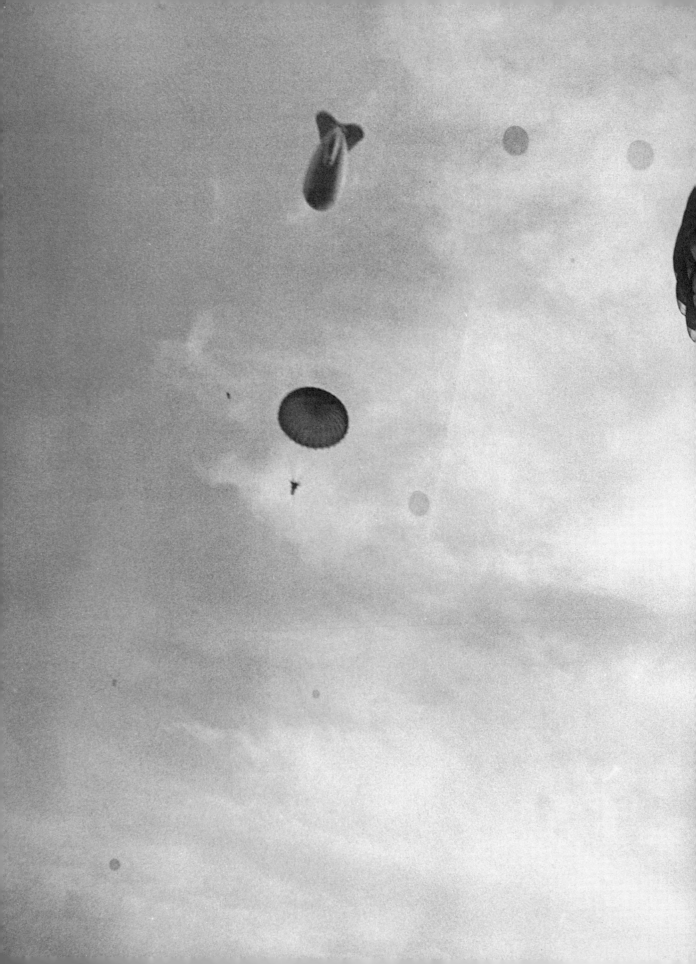

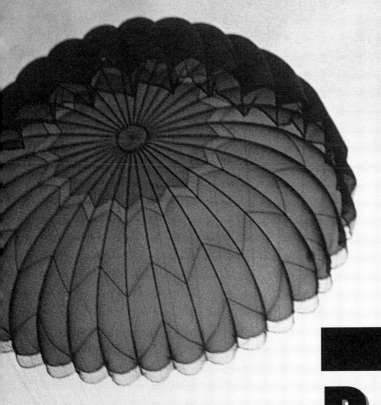

THE
PARAS
ULTIMATE
FITNESS

······························

CLAIRE GILLMAN

Hodder & Stoughton

To my husband, Nick, and my sons, Alexander and George.

Also by Claire Gillman

PARA – INSIDE THE PARACHUTE REGIMENT

Copyright © Claire Gillman 1996
The right of Claire Gillman to be identified as the Author of the Work has been
asserted by her in accordance with the Copyright, Designs and Patents Act 1988.

Exercise photographs by David Rudkin; others by Simon Walker.

First published in Great Britain by Hodder and Stoughton.
A division of Hodder Headline PLC

10 9 8 7 6 5 4 3 2 1

A CIP catalogue record for this title is available from the British Library.

ISBN 0 340 65993 9

Designed by Design/Section, Frome

Printed and bound in Great Britain by
Scotprint
Hodder and Stoughton Ltd
A Division of Hodder Headline PLC
338 Euston Road
London NW1 3BH

Acknowledgements

During my stay with the Parachute Regiment, I learned to enjoy their black sense of humour, to share their zest for life and to admire their integrity. I was teased unmercifully and have never laughed so much in my life. I now have the utmost respect for this exceptional body of men and envy them the esprit de corps that bonds them.

This is an opportunity to thank the men of The Parachute Regiment, from the highest to the lowest rank, for their help and cooperation on this project, for making it such fun and for dispelling some of the commonly held preconceptions about the military.

Singled out for a special mention in despatches are: Major Chris Kemp (PARA), Major Miles Baker (PARA) and Captain Jim Wood (APTC) for their cooperation, 'fixing' ability and advice; and Sergeant Nick Taylor (PARA) and Staff Sergeant Mark Geddes (APTC) for doing a wonderful job as models – hope you don't get too much flack from the blokes.

Thanks are also due to my husband, a former Parachute Regiment Officer, without whose inspiration and help this book would not have been possible.

Finally, without wishing to sound too much like an Oscar-winner's speech, this was a team effort. So, I'd like to thank Rachel Bond and Rowena Webb at Hodder & Stoughton for their unstinting enthusiasm, support and understanding throughout the production of this book.

Contents

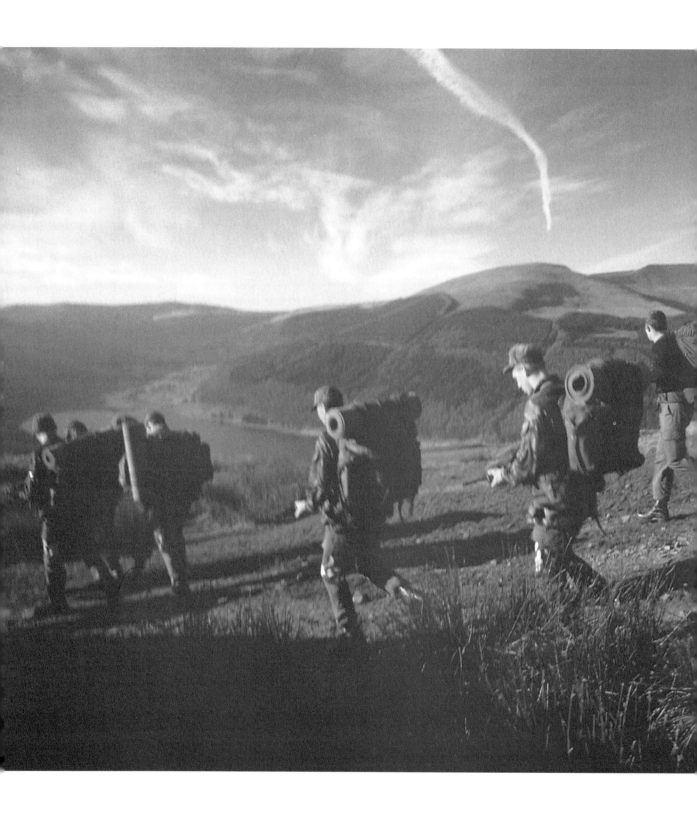

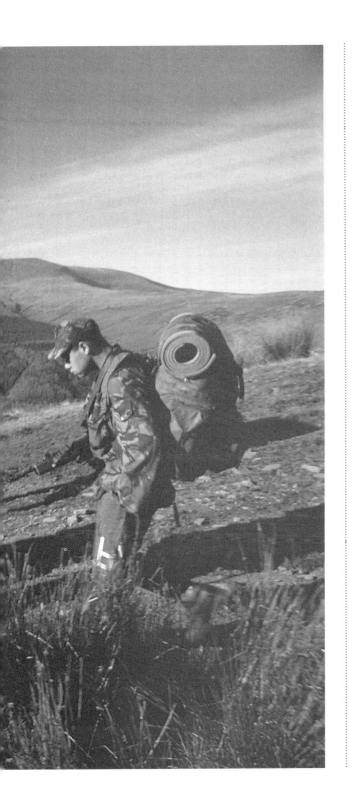

Foreword

By
**Lieutenant General
H W R Pike DSO MBE**

At the time of the Argentine invasion of the Falklands Islands in April 1982, I was the Commanding Officer of the 3rd Battalion The Parachute Regiment (3 PARA). On the Friday before Easter, we found ourselves preparing for war. On Good Friday, we sailed from Southampton on the SS Canberra. After seven weeks at sea, we landed in San Carlos Bay from assault boats with our Royal Marine comrades of 3 Commando Brigade, in order to recapture the Falklands Islands. It was winter in the South Atlantic, and the terrain was arduous.

In such circumstances, confidence is of the very essence. Confidence between commanders and their soldiers, mutual confidence within each team of soldiers, and self-confidence in each individual; confidence that 'I can do it' and that 'we can do it'. But the confidence of which I speak cannot be founded on mere 'bar-talk' or on arrogant assertions of superiority. It must be deep-rooted, substantial, enduring and resilient under the most extreme tests. Therefore, it must be born of the will to win, and this willpower can only be developed and tested through demanding physical training. This training is thus not an end in itself, though without physical fitness soldiers cannot succeed. It is the mental attitude which such training engenders, which is the real key to success on the battlefield. That tenacious spirit which is undaunted in adversity, that invincible temper of mind that overcomes misfortune, setbacks and difficulties.

This book describes the physical regime which any Parachute Regiment soldier must undergo, if he is to succeed. Through this regime, his mental qualities can also be assessed, though this is done in other ways too. I strongly commend this book to you, but must add a 'health warning'. It describes what soldiers must do, in order to join a Regiment whose members Field

Marshal Montgomery described as 'men apart'. You will notice that it is progressive, for it must change civilians into soldiers fit to undergo the sternest tests of war. But it is very demanding, and is only undertaken under the closest supervision of highly trained Instructors. Therefore, if you try to tackle anything like this on your own, unsupervised by experts, you are very likely to injure yourself needlessly and perhaps seriously. Treat the regime with respect and caution therefore, whilst enjoying the sense of achievement and well-being that comes from the physical fitness which this book can help you to achieve. And remember the confidence that it gave to those young men in the South Atlantic in 1982, and which it continues to give to their successors. It can do the same for you.

October 1995
Lieutenant General H W R Pike
DSO MBE

WARNING

If you have a medical condition, or are pregnant, you should not under any circumstances follow the programme in this book without first consulting your doctor. All guidelines, warnings and precautions should be read carefully. Neither the author, nor the publisher nor The Parachute Regiment can accept any responsibility for injuries or damage arising out of a failure to comply with the same.

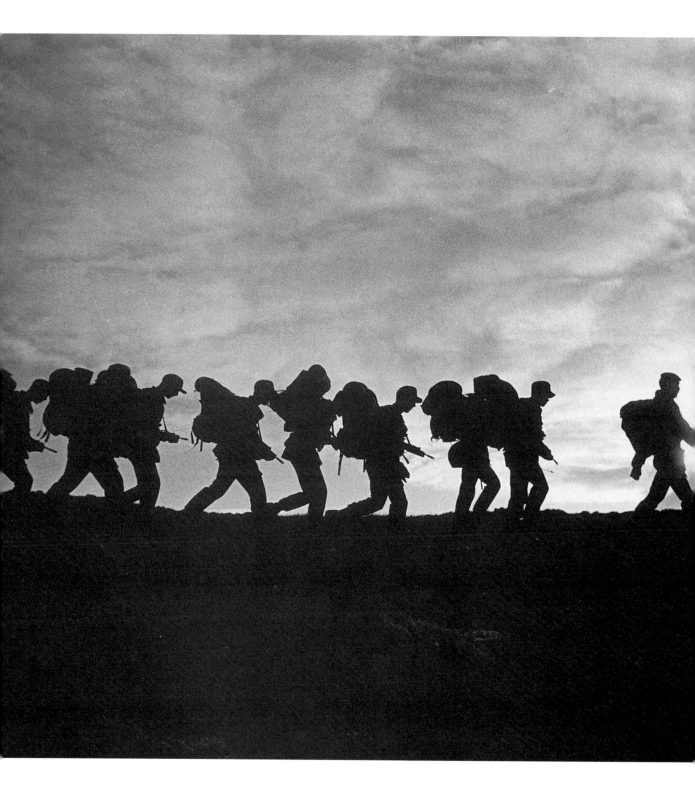

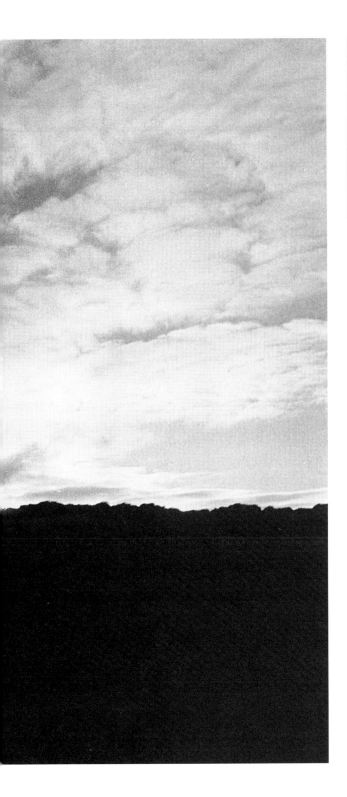

Chapter One

Utrinque Paratus - Ready For Anything

There are many different reasons why an individual embarks on a campaign to get fit. For some, it is simply the appeal of improved mental and physical well-being. For others, it is triggered by a specific reason or event – perhaps to run a marathon or to enter a sporting competition. Then there are those for whom physical fitness is a prerequisite of their vocation, such as lifeguards, sports instructors, the emergency services and the armed forces. Of the latter category, the toughest known mental and physical training is that of the army's elite, The Parachute Regiment. Their motto is Utrinque Paratus – Ready For Anything.

There is good reason for their high level of training. It has served the Regiment well in the past, particularly in 'live' situations such as the Second World War, where they earned the title 'The Red Devils' because of their ferocious fighting skills, in Suez and the partition of Cyprus and, more recently, in the Falklands and Northern Ireland.

The specific role played by a paratrooper in areas of conflict demands a high level of determination, endurance, physical strength and fitness from every serving member whatever their rank or function. The Parachute Regiment is used as a pre-emptive force, often being dropped behind enemy lines or into strategic areas such as an airfield which they must then hold, often for some days or even weeks, until support can arrive. Obviously, this requires the highest calibre of fighting soldier but, particularly in the case of being dropped behind enemy lines or in hostile territory, additional qualities are also needed.

After jumping from a low-flying aircraft, perhaps in the dark, the Para is then on his own. He has to carry any equipment he might need to survive and fight over very long distances of usually rough terrain and then be fit enough and alert enough to fight a battle against a fresh and rested enemy when he arrives at his destination. In the case of the Falklands, 2 and 3 Para marched across inhospitable, mountainous terrain carrying packs in excess of 100lbs before fighting and defeating a well dug-in enemy of vastly superior numbers (in the case of Goose Green, the Argentinian troops outnumbered the Paras 10:1). This is an illustration of the calibre of the paratrooper.

The tenacity, determination and strength of character needed to achieve such a tough objective is in no small part due to The Parachute Regiment's training programme, known as

P Company or PPS (Pre-Parachute Selection). Major C P Kemp, the officer commanding P Company at the time of writing, describes the aim of the training:

'The current aim of PPS is to test physical courage, military aptitude, fitness, endurance and determination under conditions of stress to determine whether a soldier has a self-discipline and motivation to become an airborne soldier.'

In reality, PPS achieves a great deal more. It shapes the regimental character and, because the members of the Regiment (officers, NCOs and soldiers alike) have all been through the same arduous training and tests in order to become a paratrooper (unlike any other unit of the British army), the Regiment displays a unique, cohesive esprit de corps. It is a body of men who know they are at the peak of physical fitness, that they have each proved their mettle by enduring and passing P Company and that they will not let each other down.

Ken Lukowiak who is a journalist and a former member of The Parachute Regiment says in a feature in the Guardian (June 95) on Parachute Regiment mentality:

'… Two and a half years later [after training], I ran flat out again for another mile. This time it wasn't into a training barracks but into the centre of Port Stanley. I was not alone. We were all there, two whole battalions of us, minus dead and injured, as one, together, ready to fight again. The training had paid off. In Argentina, the families of the not-so-well trained prepared for the funerals.

'So I have to say that what was done to me during training was necessary, because if it had not been taken to such extremes, I could have died. And death is very serious. I know. I've seen it. I've even caused it. And what was really done to me, and continued to be done once I joined my battalion, was that I was turned into a British Paratrooper. The toughest, fittest fighting soldier in the world.'

The young men who elect to join the Paras do so largely because they want to be a member of the toughest, most feared regiment in the British army. They have no idea just how tough it will be to achieve that goal, but when they arrive for training they are no different from you or I – they are an average 'civvy'. And, if you follow this training programme which emulates the principles as well as most of the physical aspects of the Regiment's training schedule, there is no reason why you too cannot reach peak physical fitness. This is your unique fitness challenge.

One of the key elements of The Parachute Regiment's training is their emphasis on mental toughness. It is not enough to want to be fit. You have to have the right, positive mental approach. You must develop a belief in self and in your own abilities. It is not your body that limits your performance but your mind. Often, in training, it is not the body that is ready to quit, it is the mind creating excuses why you should not go on. A paratrooper does not fail, because it never enters his head that he will not succeed. Obviously, it would be highly irresponsible to suggest that you continue to train if you have an injury. However, if you are using the discomfort of blisters as an injury excuse to quit, you have not got the right attitude. Similarly, if you

intend to cheat and not follow the programme, then this is not the training schedule for you and you are unlikely ever to achieve your goal of peak physical fitness.

It takes courage and self-belief to jump out of an aircraft flying at over 120 mph in the dark. It is that belief in their own ability which accounts for the fact that over 66% of the SAS are made up of Parachute Regiment soldiers. And it is self-belief that will get you through this training schedule.

The Parachute Regiment puts a strong emphasis on an individual's willingness and ability to help others and they rely heavily on the camaraderie that trainees develop through common hardship. This is not easy to simulate but it is widely recognised that training with a companion is much easier and more inspiring than training alone. If you can convince a friend or colleague to follow this training programme with you, it will make the tougher sessions more bearable. Obviously, it is not impossible to motivate yourself (when undertaking personal training in Battalion or for SAS selection, the Paras have to design and follow their own schedule) and, indeed, there are those who prefer to train alone but, in general, it helps to have a training partner to give each other support and encouragement.

The 16 weeks of training will get you to a level of fitness whereby you could tackle most endurance events (unless some specialist training were required) and a marathon or a triathlon would be well within your capabilities.

The test for a trainee paratrooper at the end of his 16-week training period is called P Company Test Week. He must pass this gruelling challenge in order to join the Regiment and before he is able to pass on to parachute training. The initial training has incorporated the skills that he will need as a combat soldier:

- an emphasis on lower body strength and running to prepare for approach marches carrying heavy weights;
- overall fitness and conditioning so that he is able to fight after a long, hard march; and
- upper body strength in order to carry the heavy bergen (packed rucksack) and weapons in full uniform.

As you will see, these abilities are tested to the limit during P Company Test Week. Although there is an optional test week at the end of your fitness training programme, don't worry, you won't be asked to complete the P Company test outlined below. That is a gruelling experience designed specifically for a body of men and incorporating team events. The test at the end of this book emulates the physical and mental challenges of P Company Test Week whilst using different tasks and exercises.

Test Week for the Para recruits consists of the following ten events. None of these tests taken in isolation is impossibly difficult but the cumulative physical effect and the continuous mental pressure of doing the tests one after another with inadequate rest in between make it an extremely tough ordeal. It is specifically designed to simulate the extreme mental and physical demands of parachuting in and then getting to, fighting and surviving a battle. Each test simulates an aspect of this scenario under the added pressure of a limited time span (as would be the case in a war).

Day 1

10-MILER

A 10-mile march carrying 45lbs as a formed body in 1 hr 50 mins (11 mins per mile).

TRAINASIUM

The trainasium is a high scaffolding-type structure of various heights up to 44 feet. The volunteer must show confidence in completing a number of agility tests on the structure while wearing boots and helmet. (This is a test of courage and of a recruit's ability to react to commands even when scared, as he will have to do when jumping from an aircraft into the unknown or when storming an enemy trench.)

ASSAULT COURSE

A course designed to be completed individually. The volunteer must complete a number of circuits of the course against the clock. The course is deliberately designed to prevent volunteers from getting a rhythm, to ensure they can't catch their breath and to make it as difficult as possible. (It takes strength to overcome the obstacles, and this would be required when crossing inhospitable terrain in a live situation.)

Day 2

STEEPLECHASE

The steeplechase is a 1,500m course of cross country-type obstacles to overcome at speed. It is completed twice against the clock.

THE LOG RACE

Eight men carry a large log by toggle ropes. The 2.25km course is over rough ground and steep hills and the volunteers compete against other teams. (Team work is essential in the field if cumbersome, heavy equipment is to be transported quickly to the fighting zone.)

MILLING

Milling takes the form of a one-minute round wearing heavy 18oz boxing gloves. Each volunteer is matched against an opponent of similar size and weight. Headguards are worn and it is a round of controlled aggression. (In the British army, milling is only used in SAS and Parachute Regiment selection.)

Day 3

APPROACH MARCH

An 18-mile approach march over rugged hill terrain is completed by squads in 4 hrs 30 mins carrying 45lbs plus weapon in full kit.

Day 4

12-MILE MARCH

A 12-mile march over rolling hills is completed by squads in 2 hrs 35 mins carrying 45lbs. Immediately followed by:

10KM BATTLE MARCH

After a mere 30-minute stop following the 12-mile march, the volunteers complete a 10km battle march as a formed body in 1 hr 8 mins.

Day 5

STRETCHER RACE

The stretcher race is a team event carrying a 140lbs metal stretcher on a 6-mile course over rough and undulating terrain (a close approximation of evacuating wounded colleagues from a battle scene).

Each event is marked out of 10 with the exception of the trainasium which is a straight pass or fail – refuse a section and you have failed the whole course. The pass mark is 55 which represents 'strong sustained effort throughout test week' (P Company charter). The fail mark is 50 and those who score between these limits lie in the discussion bracket, when judgement is applied.

There is no fixed number who have to pass. If volunteers do not make the grade then they simply have to try again, and the pass rate from courses has been known to fall as low as 29%. The Parachute Regiment will not compromise its standards and only wants the fittest men with the right mental approach.

Incidentally, if like myself, a march conjures up a walking pace to you, think again. A march is conducted at a jogging or running pace and on many occasions during my stay with the Paras, I was forced to jump into the support land rover because I couldn't keep up with the main body of men. Hence, marches are retitled runs in the training schedule.

In order to attain your personal goal of completing the programme in this book, you will need good preparation, the right equipment and plenty of determination. Bear in mind The Parachute Regiment motto, Ready for Anything, and then anything is achievable.

Having completed your Paras Ultimate Fitness Training Programme, you will be extremely fit (and probably a lot thinner!). What you choose to do with your new-found level of fitness is purely down to the individual. You will undoubtedly be enjoying the heightened sense of well-being, the new levels of energy and the sharper mind that fitness brings with it. To maintain this high level of fitness requires a continued commitment to training, but you can choose the level of fitness and degree of effort to put in that suit your lifestyle and domestic/working commitments (see Chapter 8 Maintaining Fitness).

For the successful recruits moving in to Battalion, fitness becomes an integral part of their working lives. It is almost a by-product of their way of life rather than something they have to maintain or seek to achieve. After passing P Company, and once he has earned his wings, a Para joins his Battalion where his fitness, attitude and soldiering skills are honed and tested. During the course of his working day, he will regularly run distances varying from 6 to 18 miles, sometimes at speed and sometimes with heavy weights in the bergen. (It has been known for Battalions to run 50 miles with weight.) A trick often played on

new-comers is secretly to fill their bergen with rocks after it has been weighed at the required weight. The unsuspecting victim wonders why he is finding the going so tough!

On exercise, where the Para could be living rough in the field for up to two weeks in different parts of the world, with varying and often hostile climates, great distances can be covered during the exercise and, since the men are self-supporting, enormous weight has to be carried. It is not unusual for men to carry bergens of 80–100lbs and more, in addition to their personal weapon of at least 9lbs, and those of the Support Company (responsible for heavy weapons such as mortars, anti-tank weapons etc.) are carrying considerably more. Obviously, exercise sessions and physical training are an essential feature of their daily lives. However, the robustness of their general work and the relentlessness of the physical demands placed upon them means that the Paras' strength lies in their endurance and toughness.

As you read these introductory chapters, your personal goal is yet to be reached and it is a daunting challenge.

Yet, I can assure you, once attained, the feeling of walking 10 feet tall is well worth the effort.

How To Use This Book

In Chapter 2, there is a pre-exercise questionnaire (p. 27). This must be satisfactorily completed before embarking on the fitness assessment test which appears in the same chapter (p. 26).

Once you have met the minimum fitness requirements of the assessment test, you then qualify to start the programme. You will find advice on the equipment needed throughout your training in Chapter 3 and tips on how to prepare mentally for this challenge in Chapter 4. Useful pointers on dealing with injuries, and advice on nutrition for your training schedule can be found in Chapters 5 and 6.

Having read and digested all this information, you are then ready to embark on The Paras Ultimate Fitness Training Programme in Chapter 7. At the end of that chapter you will find log tables which you can fill in as you progress through the schedule. These provide a helpful and interesting record of your improved fitness levels.

I am sure you are keen to get started on the training programme but it is imperative that you read all the relevant chapters and undergo the assessments before embarking on the programme. This precaution is for very sound health and safety reasons.

Finally, once you have achieved your goal and completed the programme, you will find advice on maintaining your new-found levels of fitness in Chapter 8.

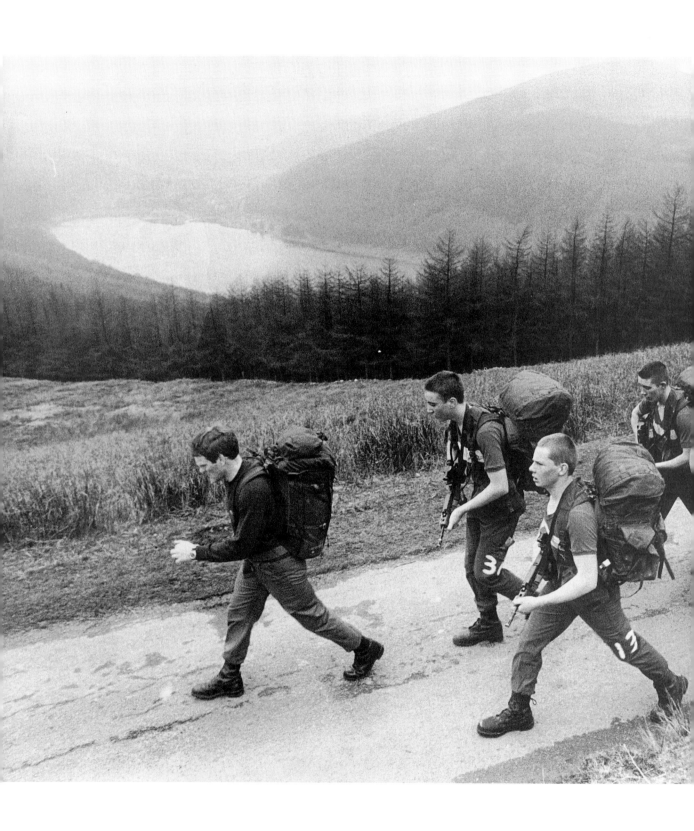

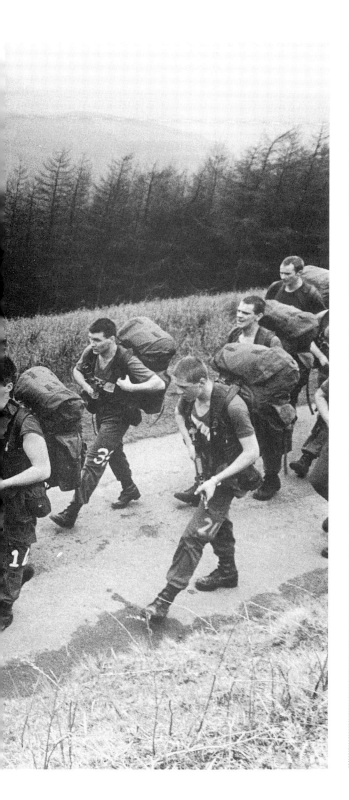

Chapter Two

Are You Fighting Fit?

• •

A nybody wishing to join the British army undergoes a medical examination before being recruited. This is a precautionary measure designed to safeguard the recruit's health and one that we will also adhere to on this training programme.

How Fit Are You?

'Exercise has long been shown to give rise to an enhanced sense of well-being and an increased capacity for physical activity which enriches practical involvement in daily life. This happens because, with exercise, there are marked physiological improvements in the normal function of many body systems.'

Fentem & Bassey 1978

If you complete The Paras Ultimate Fitness you will experience the benefits of better health and a greater sense of well-being. These are manifested in the following improvements in levels of physical fitness:

- reduction in obesity;
- prevention of coronary heart disease;
- fewer health problems in old age;
- improvements in physical health.

Mentally, the benefits include:

- increased self-confidence;
- increased assertiveness;
- greater self-awareness; and
- better concentration levels.

However, such benefits can only be achieved if all the components of physical fitness are improved. Namely:

- cardio-respiratory fitness (stamina, endurance, aerobic fitness);
- strength;
- local muscular endurance;
- flexibility; and
- motor fitness (agility, balance, coordination, power, speed and reaction time).

Training for entry to the Regiment and The Parachute Regiment Ultimate Fitness Training Programme are both specifically designed to incorporate each of these aspects of physical fitness. However, we do not all start out equal in the physical fitness stakes. Each individual responds differently to exercise and has a different potential for improvement. There are many factors which affect our optimum fitness levels, some of which we cannot alter such as heredity, sex, body type, age and, to some degree, state of health. Others, such as diet and lifestyle, are areas which we can influence (see Chapter 6).

Smoking

As a smoker, you run a far greater risk of heart disease and lung cancer. Smokers are also at a disadvantage when exercising because they require more oxygen to achieve the same performance as a non-smoker. Smokers may find that in the initial stages of training, the running and stamina exercises are somewhat harder.

Alcohol

It is recommended that you consume only moderate amounts of alcohol while following The Parachute Regiment Ultimate Fitness Training Programme. Paras are not known for their abstinence when it comes to alcohol but this is normally once they have joined their Battalion and enjoy peak physical fitness. Recruits don't get much opportunity to go drinking and it is probably for good reason – training with a hangover is neither fun nor effective.

Drugs

The debilitating effects of drugs are well documented and it is only necessary to mention here that a Para would automatically be dismissed from the army if caught taking drugs.

The Paras Ultimate Fitness is designed for men. However, if the minimum entry level requirements are achieved, there is no reason why a woman cannot follow this programme. The same cautionary principles apply for both men and women – if you are in pain or feel unwell, do not continue. If you are pregnant, do not attempt to undertake this programme under any circumstances.

Medical Condition

It is always advisable to see your doctor before starting a strenuous training programme but if you answer Yes to any of the questions in the pre-exercise questionnaire on p. 27, then you should definitely see your GP before embarking on any form of exercise. If you answer No to all the questions, you have a reasonable assurance of your suitability for a graduated exercise programme. You can now embark on the following fitness assessment test to find out just how fit or otherwise you really are.

Fitness Assessment Test

There are numerous ways to measure fitness levels. For the purposes of this book, we will look at one basic method. If you achieve timings within the bracket of average or above in the assessment table on p. 26, then you are sufficiently fit to start The Paras Ultimate Fitness Programme. If not, some moderate exercises are suggested later in this chapter which will soon get you to a standard at which you can start the programme. Follow these gentle exercises for several weeks and then retake the assessment test.

FITNESS ASSESSMENT TEST

(Not to be attempted until Pre-exercise Questionnaire successfully completed)

Distance	(time in minutes)			
	Very Good	Good	Average	Below Average
1 mile	3.45–5	5–6	6–7	8–10
4 mile	20–24	24–28	28–32	32–26
6 mile	30–33	33–35	35–38	38–42
8 mile	48–50	50–55	55–60	60–65
10 miles	60–62	62–70	70–80	80–90

You will need running/training shoes, a track suit to warm up in, shorts and a T-shirt for the actual run and a stopwatch or a watch with an accurate second-hand. For the test, you must select a route with the distance clearly marked. Obviously, access to a running track may be an advantage for this.

Before starting your run, follow the warm-up routine as outlined on p. 35-45.

The table above gives test times (in minutes) for a one-mile run and for longer distances. These are similar to the standards required of Parachute Regiment soldiers. Incidentally, take note that the runs include various gradients.

The minimum standard to pass the army's Basic Fitness Test (BFT) is 10 mins 30 secs for a 1.5 mile run. To attend the Parachute Regiment PPS Course (after 5 weeks of training), the minimum standard is 9 mins 30 secs for the 1.5 mile run.

The Parachute Regiment also uses the bleep test. This test against the clock initially appears innocuous, but it gets progressively tougher and becomes a hard grind. It varies from other measurements of fitness in that you give up when you want to or feel you have to – it is therefore also a measure of mental toughness. It is a shuttle-run test whereby you have to run a set distance, turn and run back again within a certain time. The pace starts

PRE-EXERCISE QUESTIONNAIRE

		YES	NO
1.	Has your GP ever said you have heart disease, high blood pressure or any other cardiovascular problem?	❏	❏
2.	Is there a history of heart disease in your family?	❏	❏
3.	Do you ever have pains in your heart and chest, especially associated with minimal effort?	❏	❏
4.	Do you often get headaches, feel faint or dizzy?	❏	❏
5.	Do you suffer from pain or limited movement in any joints, which has been aggravated by exercise or might be made worse with exercise?	❏	❏
6.	Are you taking drugs/medication at the moment or recuperating from a recent illness or operation?	❏	❏
7.	Are you unaccustomed to exercise and aged over 35?	❏	❏
8.	Do you have any other medical condition which you think may affect your ability to participate in exercise?	❏	❏

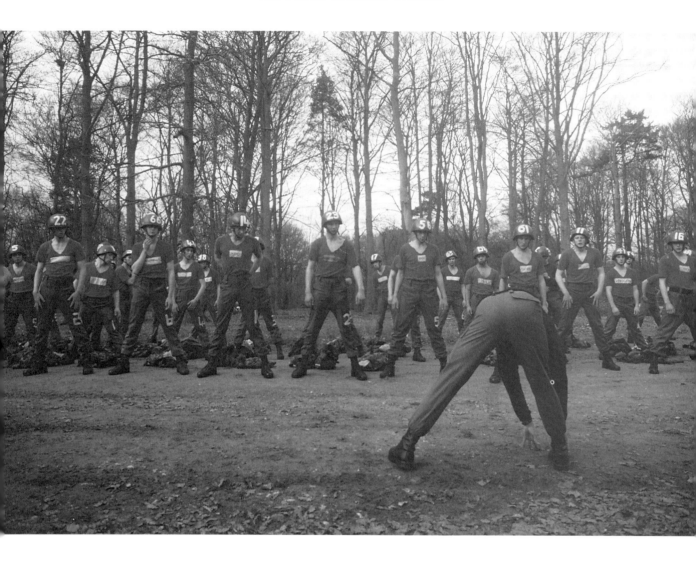

quite leisurely and it progresses level by level until you are sprinting up and down the track.

There are commercially produced versions of the bleep test. The Multistage Fitness Test is one of the best. It consists of a high-quality audio cassette containing full instructions and timing indicators for the test, two markers to be placed 20m apart, together with a 12-page explanatory booklet. It is available from The National Coaching Foundation, 4 College Close, Beckett Park, Leeds LS6 3QH.

Remember: if you are not up to the minimum fitness requirements, which is the Average column in the table above, do not start the programme. It is not worth cheating as you could injure yourself or seriously damage your health. It is far more sensible to take a little longer in preparation for the training.

Here are some ways to gently raise your fitness standard prior to starting The Paras Ultimate Fitness Training Programme.

Complete a minimum of three sessions a week of one hour duration (including warm-up and cool-down) selecting from activities such as jogging, cycling, swimming, flexibility exercises, and the following elements of circuit training (see pages 78-88): press-ups, sit-ups, step-ups, leg lifts. Simply do one set of 10 repetitions for each exercise.

Make sure that you start slowly and gently, never exceeding what feels comfortable and then gradually increase the amount of effort you put in, for example the number of lengths swum, the distance jogged or cycled, the number of repetitions of circuit elements. After several weeks, retry the fitness assessment test.

Monitoring Progress

As well as sporadically doing the run tests to see how your fitness is improving throughout the programme, a useful and quick guide to progress is to monitor your pulse.

The pulse can be located and measured either at the main artery on the side of the neck, just below the jaw, or on the inside of the wrist in line with the thumb. Simply use the first two fingers of one hand to count the number of beats over a certain period. Obviously a full minute gives the most accurate reading but you can take it over 30 seconds and double it, over 15 seconds and multiply by 4, or over 10 seconds and multiply by 6.

When you wake in the morning after a full night's sleep, take your pulse rate over one minute to determine your resting pulse rate. Do this for three days and take the average as your resting rate. During the training schedule, if the resting rate is more than ten beats per minute higher than your average, perhaps you are over-exerting yourself and you should rest that day and consider training the next day. However, your pulse rate during a normal morning's activity, at work for instance, should be about ten beats per minute higher than your resting rate.

During training, the aim is to get your pulse rate up to 60–85% of your Maximum Heart Rate (MHR). To calculate your MHR, simply deduct your age in years from 220. Initially, you should not aim to train at levels about 75% of MHR. However, if you do not achieve this rate for more than 20 minutes at least three times a week, you are not working aerobically and therefore are not actually achieving your training capacity.

As a guideline to fitness, the resting pulse rate of an average adult male, awake but at rest, is between 60–80 beats per minute (on average, 71 beats per minute). A woman's rate is slightly higher at about 80 beats per minute. As your fitness level increases, these figures will probably drop by anything up to ten beats per minute, giving a resting pulse rate of around 60 during normal activity and a waking pulse rate of about 52 beats per minute.

All recruits who join the army follow the same initial fitness training at Lichfield with the Army Physical Training Instructors or PT Busters. However, those who are being groomed for The Parachute Regiment have to achieve higher entry levels of fitness before being accepted on the Pre-Parachute Selection (PPS) training at Catterick (after 5 weeks at Lichfield). For example, as previously mentioned, the army-wide standard for a BFT (Basic Fitness Test) is to complete the 1.5 mile run in under 10 mins 30 secs; the standard required for The Parachute Regiment is a full minute less than that at 9 mins 30 secs. Following this programme, you should be achieving under 10 minutes in the first 5 weeks and under 9 mins 30 secs after the first 10 weeks of your training.

On joining the army, all recruits are expected to take and pass a Military Swim Test comprising treading water for 2 mins followed by four lengths of a 25m pool using any stroke except back stroke. Therefore, the ability to swim is essential to becoming a Para. However, for the purpose of following this training schedule, it is not a prerequisite and, if necessary, the swimming sessions can be replaced with some other aerobic fitness session for all-round conditioning such as cycling, or high- or low-impact aerobics (see Chapter 8, Maintaining Fitness).

Having passed the Fitness Assessment Test, it is now time to get the necessary equipment and your thoughts together, before starting The Paras Ultimate Fitness Training Programme.

Body Type

There are three basic body types:

- Ectomorph: long and lean with narrow shoulders and hips.
- Mesomorph: strong and muscular with broad shoulders and narrow hips.
- Endomorph: short with wide rounded hips, limbs and face.

Although ectomorphs are known for their natural aptitude as long-distance runners and mesomorphs tend to be good at carrying weight, each category has some advantages to offer. Paras come in all shapes and sizes and body type alone should not affect your ability to undergo this training.

Irrespective of your body type, it is highly probable that you will lose weight or inches when following The Paras Ultimate Fitness Training Programme. Don't be surprised if you do, even if you weren't overweight to start with – this is a strenuous programme which uses a lot of energy!

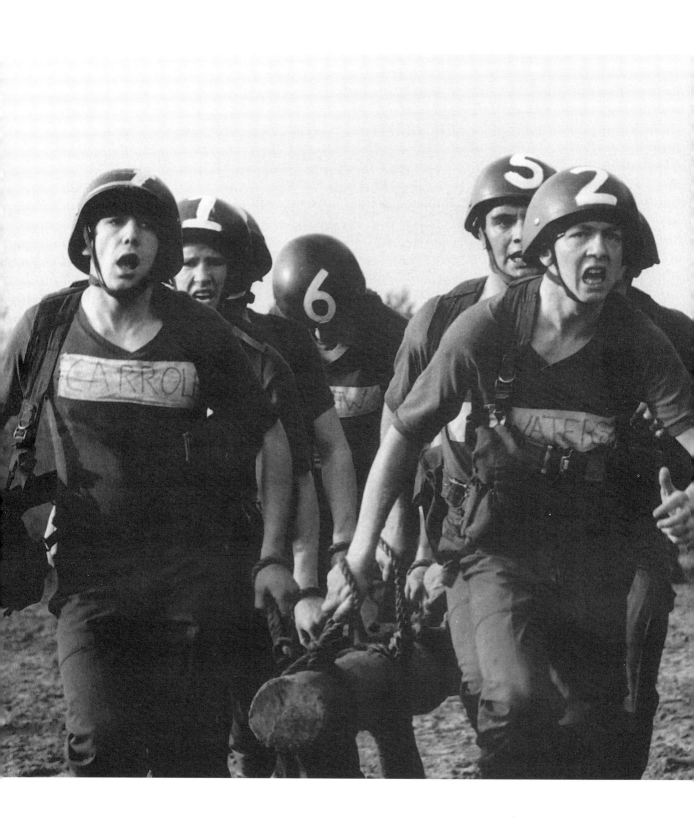

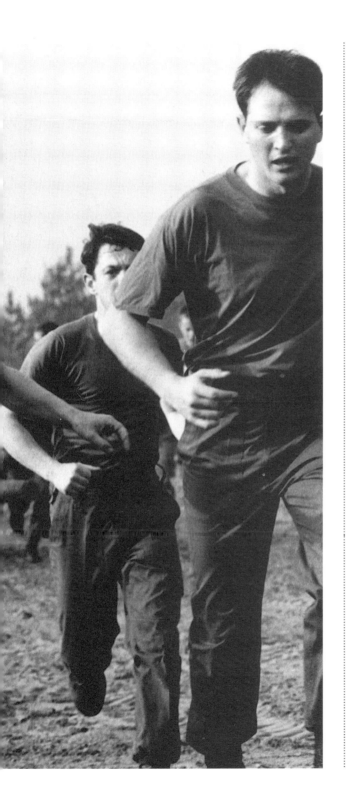

Chapter Three

Preparation

● ●

Before embarking on The Paras Ultimate Fitness Training Programme, check the equipment you will need for the next 16 weeks.

It is not necessary to go out and spend a fortune on new equipment. However, if you are serious about getting fit and maintaining fitness, then a small investment in good kit is worthwhile. Initially, it may be worth borrowing equipment from friends until you are certain you want to continue with the fitness quest. Similarly, access to a gym or running track would be very useful but fitness centres make their money out of those who join in a rare moment of enthusiasm, use the facilities exhaustively for several weeks and never come back again. So be warned.

Equipment you will need

1. Buy a local OS 1:50,000 map or better still, a 1:25,000 which shows footpaths, and then explore your local area. Work out circular routes and, if you have the help of your family or friends with a car, a few linear ones. Ask to be taken to the start point and run home rather than collected at the end of a run. Psychologically it is better. For the BFT, the Paras always walk out to the start and run back to camp as fast as they can.

2. Training/running shoes. Good quality running shoes are essential for this programme which puts emphasis on high-mileage running training. Therefore, if you don't already have a good pair of trainers, it's worth going to a specialist running shop or athletics store to buy a new pair. If you already run, take an old pair with you for the assistant to check wear. £50–60 should get you a decent pair of running shoes but a good rule of thumb is to buy the best you can afford.

3. Basic training kit comprises:
   - Numerous T-shirts and vests.
   - Shorts.
   - Track tops and bottoms.
   - Sports socks.
   - Good watch with a second hand and/or a stopwatch.
   - If training in poor weather, you will also need woolly hat and gloves.
   - For early morning, evening and night-time running, invest in a fluorescent vest and reflective arm and ankle bands.
   - Whatever the time of year, you will need some waterproof clothing. A breathable fabric top with hood and trousers are recommended.

4. Daypack. Whether you intend to train with weight or not, get one with chest and waist straps which fits comfortably and wear it in. On long runs, carry fluid, either hot or cold depending on the weather, sweets and chocolate, map, compass, a safety blanket and basic first aid kit in case of injury, and spare socks.

5. Access to a bicycle, swimming pool, skipping rope, gymnasium or athletics track is useful.

You will see from the training schedule that, for many of the marches/runs, the recruits train in full military kit i.e. boots, bergens (large rucksacks packed with weight), helmets and weapon (9lbs). Although the word 'march' conjures up a walk, this is not usually the case, and the pace is that of a slow to moderate run. It is therefore recommended that you always train in running/training shoes as there is no merit for the civilian in wearing boots. However, if you prefer to wear a lightweight fell boot/running shoe with ankle support for some of the 'marches' over rough terrain, that is purely a matter of personal choice.

The same holds true for training with weight on your back. For The Parachute Regiment, the training involves progressively heavier weight for good reason as it prepares the men for a specific function (see Chapter 1). However, there is no documentary evidence that training with weight will improve fitness. It is worth taking a backpack to carry your essential kit (see above) but it is not recommended that you follow the load bearing of the Paras. This information is included in the schedule simply for interest.

However, if you are determined to mirror the Para training as closely as possible and to carry similar weights, then make sure that you have a well-fitting rucksack and watch out for 'bergen burns' (rubbing raw of the skin on the back) as this can slow up your progress.

There are certain prerequisites of every training session, whether it be running, leisure activity or circuit training. These are that you always allow time for warming up and cooling down, and that you do not neglect the rest days in your training programme – they are as essential as the training itself.

Warm-up

The need for warming up before taking exercise cannot be overstressed. Its purpose is:

- to prepare the body for activity (our bodily systems take time to adapt to the increased demands of exercise);
- to maximise performance (there is some evidence to suggest that a suitable warm-up period can lead to improvements of up to 20% in flexibility test ratings); and

- to avoid the possibility of suffering muscular soreness and injury.

The components of a good warm-up should comprise:

- exercises to gradually raise the heart rate and increase the body temperature;
- mobilising exercises, incorporating gentle, rhythmic movements to take the various joints of the body through their full range of normal movement;
- easy stretching exercises; and
- exercises to bring your heart rate up to workout level.

Only start the stretching exercises once the body temperature has been raised and the joints fully mobilised.

There are no clear-cut guidelines as to the duration of the warm-up period but you should allow a minimum of 10 minutes to warm up before every training session and, in some cases, up to 30 minutes. Obviously, in colder conditions and early in the morning, more time should be allowed. Similarly, if the exercise session which follows is going to be very demanding or of a longer duration, then a longer period of warm-up is required.

The following warm-up exercises should prepare your body for the extra stresses of your training routine. All movements should be carried out at least 10 times, slowly and smoothly at first so that the muscles and joints have time to adapt to the new tensions placed upon them. Finally, repeat the exercises again a minimum of 10 times with more vigour, but with the movements remaining smooth and comfortable. When stretching, do not strain or bounce – approach the point of maximum stretch slowly and then hold the position for 30–60 seconds. Slowly return to a relaxed position.

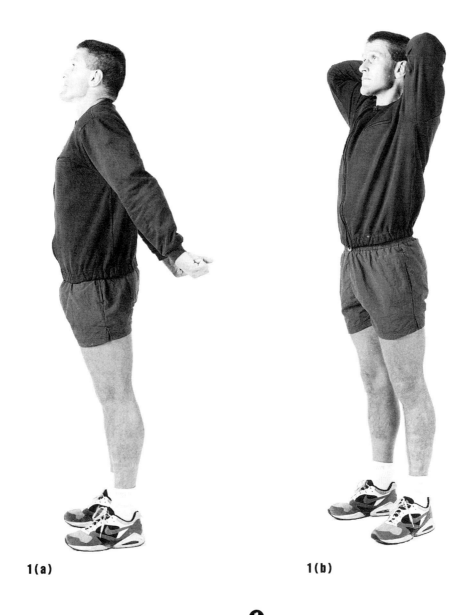

1(a)   1(b)

❶

(a) Arms straight, clench fists and push slightly behind body.
(b) Swing arms forward, over head and bend elbows at full extent of swing, hands reaching down behind head.

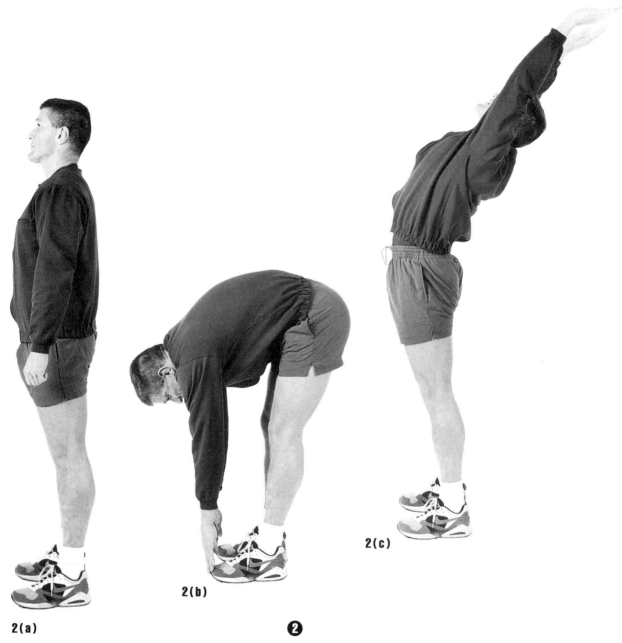

2(a)

2(b)

2(c)

❷

(a) Stand straight.

(b) As you bend your trunk forward, slide hands down the front of your legs. Keep legs straight but do not overstrain.

(c) Return to standing and arch back, arms reaching out above head.

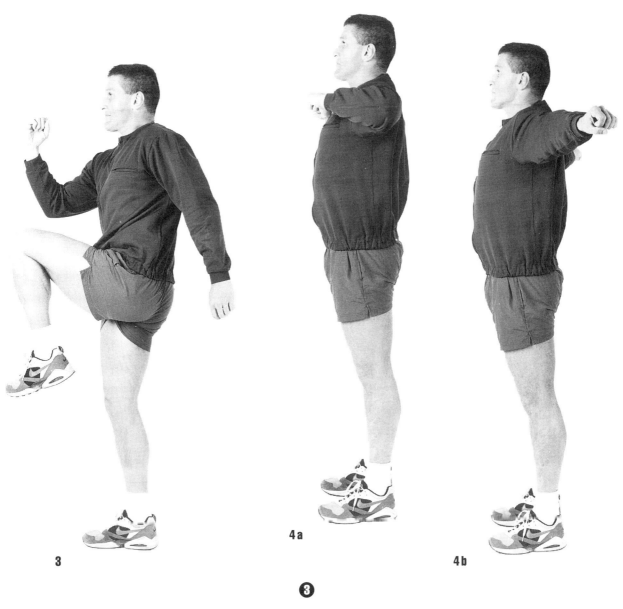

3

4a

4b

❸

Alternate raising the knee towards the chest, with the opposite arm forward.

❹

(a) Bend arms horizontally at elbows at shoulder height. Gently press bent arms back once.

(b) Then press straight arms back once at the same height.

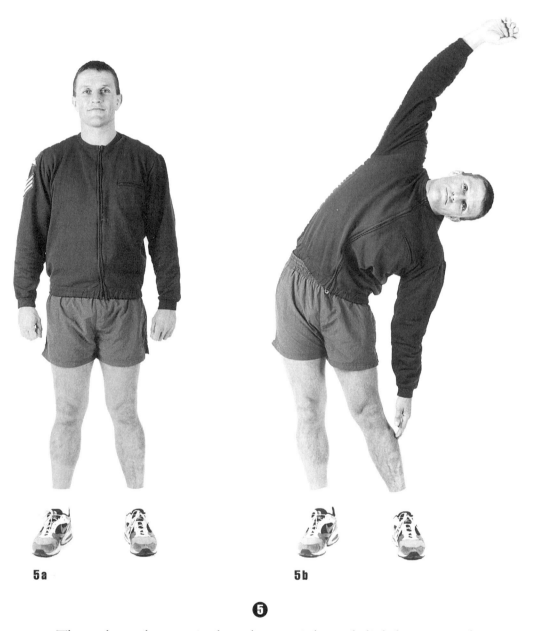

5a   **5b**

❺

(a) Throughout the exercise keep legs straight and slightly apart with feet flat on the floor.

(b) Bend on alternate sides with hand sliding down the outside of the leg. The opposite arm reaches over head.

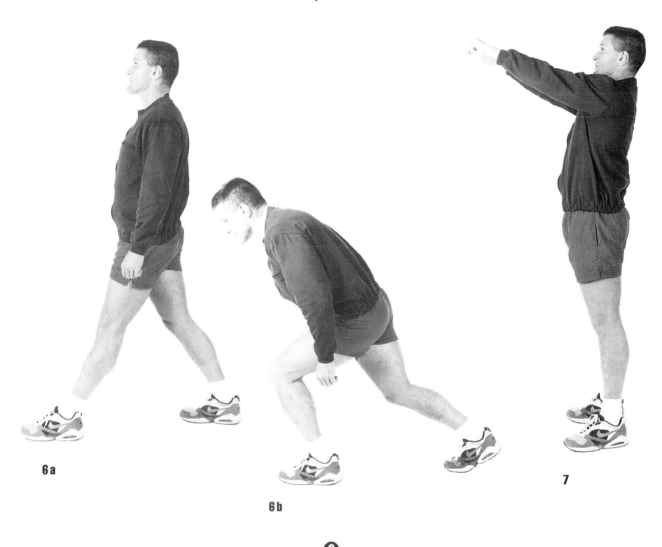

6a

6b

7

6

(a) Take a stride forward.

(b) Lower yourself forward until the leading knee is over your leading foot. Return smoothly to start position. Pivot round and repeat with the opposite leg leading.

7

Circle your arms fully, first forward and then backward. Keep arms close to the head during inward circle.

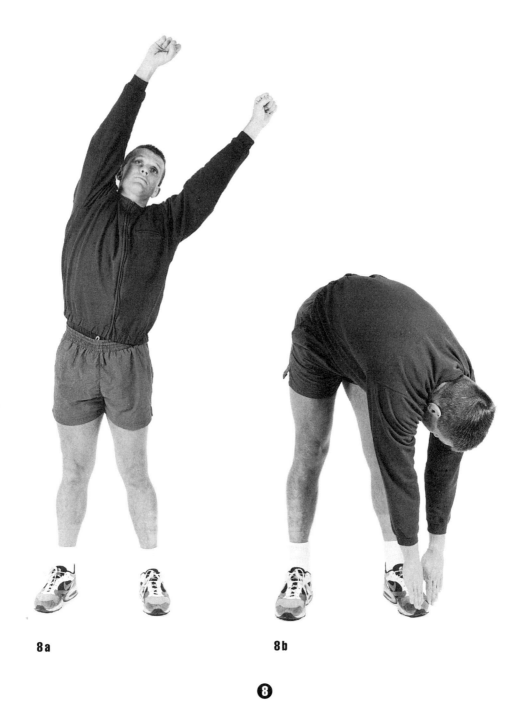

8a

8b

❽

(a) With legs astride, extend arms.

(b+c) Circle trunk fully. Keep legs straight throughout.

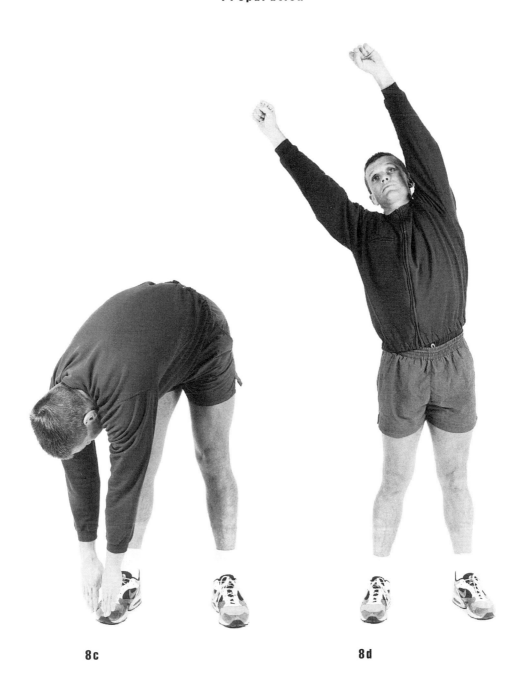

8c   8d

(d) Arch back whilst passing through upright position. Circle alternately left and right.

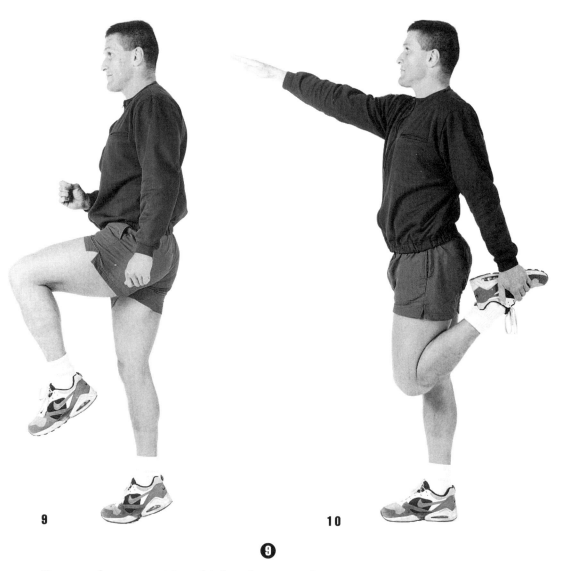

9

10

❾

Run on the spot, raising thigh to horizontal position (ten repetitions on each leg).

❿

Standing on your right leg, reach back and grasp left ankle with left hand. Pull ankle back (not to the side) until you feel the stretch in the front of the thigh. Repeat with the right leg.

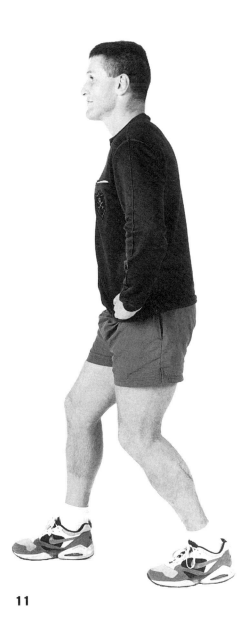

11

⑪

With hands on hips, lean your body slightly forward. Put right leg forward, keeping left heel on the ground until you feel hamstring and calf being stretched. Then bend left knee slightly and stretch the Achilles tendon. Repeat with other leg.

Cool-down

Just as vital as the warm-up period, is a cool-down after the main period of activity is completed. The body needs to make numerous adaptations before its systems return to their normal pre-exercise levels and anything we can do to help this recovery process is useful (see Chapter 6, Nutrition For Training).

Always keep warm while going through the cool-down process to avoid the risk of injury. Examples of ways to lower the pulse and cool down include gentle jogging, skipping and walking, gradually decreasing in intensity, and rhythmic flowing exercises such as arm swings, or knee bends. You can even repeat some of the exercises used in the mobilising stage of the warm-up. Take anywhere between 5 and 10 minutes to cool down. Remember, after an exercise session, showers or baths should be warm rather than hot, and sauna and steam baths are not advisable.

Rest

It is imperative to take adequate rest periods. The training sessions are designed to be carried out within a 7-day week in the order presented. Irrespective of your other commitments, never do more than one session per day and make sure you have adequate rest between training sessions i.e. don't try and cram all your training into the weekend. It may be hard to force yourself to go out for a run after a difficult day at work but that's part of the self-discipline of training. (Although the programme is progressively designed to build fitness over 16 weeks, should you want to repeat a week for any reason this is permissible.)

There are also very good physiological reasons why the programme is designed as it is. The human body is infinitely adaptable – its capabilities are not fixed. If an exercise programme is well devised and adhered to, only unavoidable illnesses or injuries can prevent your progress towards a fitter and healthier state of being. However, once you have achieved a high level of physical fitness, the benefits gained can only be maintained by regular activity – but more of that later (see Chapter 8, Maintaining Fitness).

Once the basic physiological theory of exercise is grasped, the importance of following a programme of exercise and resting sufficiently becomes clear. The principles of improved fitness are straightforward. In order to achieve greater fitness, you must stress the body's systems to a higher level than that to which they are normally subjected i.e. passing beyond a certain critical threshold to bring about the desired adaptation. If this threshold is not exceeded, no improvement will occur. During a training session, there is a breakdown of the tissue reserves and cell constituents and the accumulation of 'fatigue' by-products. During the recovery or rest period, the body replaces more than was lost and this excessive replacement temporarily enhances the body's fitness level. This gain will be lost, however, if no further exercise is undertaken. So, if we are to enhance our fitness levels, exercise must be planned and scheduled so that fitness levels continue to improve. Hence the structure of The Parachute Regiment Ultimate Fitness Training Programme.

It is a great temptation when first starting a fitness programme to be over-enthusiastic in the early stages and to overtrain. This is counter-productive. You are likely to end up in pain and discomfort, severely fatigued and more prone to injury. It is at this stage that many would-be fitness enthusiasts drop out. It is far more effective to build up your level of work intensity over a period of time and that is why The Parachute Regiment Ultimate Fitness Training Programme is so devised. Unfortunately, there are no short cuts to getting fit! It takes determination, persistence and hard work.

'It should be appreciated that during exercise the musculo-skeletal system of the body is subjected to a considerable amount of mechanical stress which inevitably results in micro-trauma (mechanical fatigue) to the musculo-skeletal tissues, especially muscle, blood vessels and connective tissues. Given adequate rest, the tissues will not only heal but also adapt (remodel) their structures over time in order to more readily withstand the stress imposed during exercise. However, when rest periods are inadequate, the fatigue process outpaces the remodelling process such that microtrauma gradually accumulate and eventually result in what is termed a chronic or overuse injury.'

Sperryn 1983

The Golden Rules of Training

1. *USE GOOD KIT, PARTICULARLY FOR FEET.*

   If buying new footwear or equipment, take advice from a specialist shop and buy the best you can afford for your particular requirements. Don't forget to get good socks as well.

2. *ALWAYS WARM UP AND COOL DOWN.*

3. *VARY YOUR TRAINING.*

   Avoid boredom by changing routes and occasionally substituting a different but commensurate form of training.

4. *KEEP A LOG/DIARY OF YOUR TRAINING.*

   Use the sheets provided (see end of Chapter 7) or make your own to note the time of day of your runs, the type of training, the time you spent out, etc. It makes fascinating reading in months to come. And don't cheat – your progress will be fast enough without embellishing the records!

5. *NEVER OVERDO YOUR TRAINING.*

   Ease off if you are very tired and make sure you get the necessary rest periods between training sessions.

6. *NEVER TRAIN IF YOU HAVE A TEMPERATURE.*

   Severe exertion when you have a temperature puts an unnecessary strain on the heart and is very unwise.

7. *WEAR WHITE OR REFLECTIVE CLOTHING IF RUNNING AT NIGHT.*

   This is particularly important if you are running on pavements rather than using a running/training track.

8. *NEVER RUN OR TRAIN THROUGH AN INJURY.*

   If you are satisfied that it is a genuine injury, stop training immediately and treat (see Chapter 5, Dealing With Injuries). Return to the schedule only once you have fully recovered, and restart at a level some weeks before the point at which you stopped.

9. *DO NOT TRAIN IF YOU HAVE FLU, A FEVERISH COLD OR A TUMMY BUG.*

10. *THE PARAS HAVE A SAYING: 'GOD LOVES THE INFANTRY'.*

    This basically means, whatever the weather you've got to get out there and do it. Don't postpone a session because of the rain or sessions will start to back up and the careful balance of your training schedule will be lost.

11. *YOU MUST REPLACE FLUIDS LOST IN SWEAT.*

    Drink plenty of fluids after training and during races, otherwise your body becomes dehydrated and less efficient.

12. *ONCE STARTED, DON'T CHANGE YOUR EXERCISE SESSION.*

    If you start modifying on a good day, psychologically you are more likely to cut corners on a bad day. Plan it and do it.

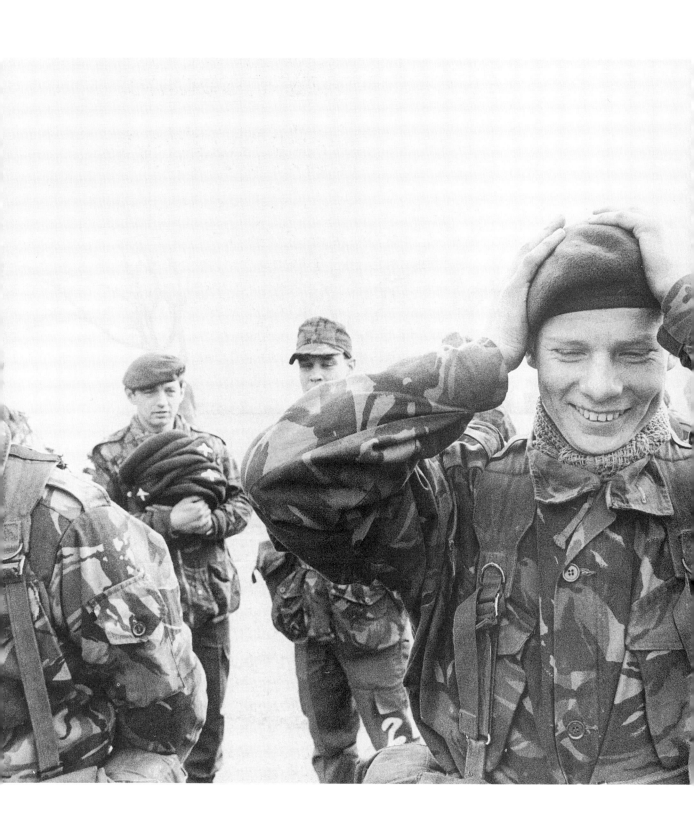

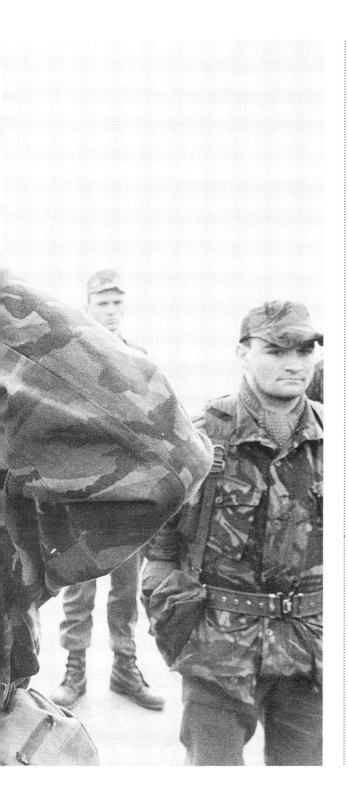

Chapter Four

Motivation

•••••••••••••••••••••••

The Paras use the lure of the elusive red beret and its reputation to great effect. Recruits desperately want to belong to and be part of this elite group of men. The training staff maintain a distance and deliberately keep a superior approach to non-Paras and to recruits (Joes) to heighten the effect of wanting to be part of the Regiment. Wanting something so badly is a great motivator and can overcome many of the hardships of strenuous physical training. The powerful influence of the red beret continues once men have earned their wings and are in Battalion. It is worn with immense pride. I have personally witnessed exhausted recruits at the end of P Company Test Week grow an inch with glowing pride as the Red Beret is placed on their heads.

One seasoned sergeant, not normally given to flights of fancy, confided that when the going gets tough in his personal training, he dons his red beret. He says:

'When I put the beret on my head, I can keep going. There is something mystical about the beret.'

The beret obviously gives him a psychological boost because it is symbolic of so much to him.

It doesn't matter what it is that motivates you. In the case of the recruits, the motivating goal is the cachet of joining The Parachute Regiment. For you, it could be the objective of finishing the London Marathon or a half marathon, completing a triathlon or being able to run a sub-4-minute mile. Whatever it is that you hope to achieve, you have got to want it badly enough to put yourself through some hard training. Choose a goal that is difficult but not impossible and something that is important to you, no matter how strange it may seem to others. After all, they are going to think you mad for doing this anyway.

Although the main target you set yourself at the start of this programme is your ultimate goal, you can set yourself smaller hurdles to overcome during training as this helps get you to the end objective. For example, aim to complete the 5-mile run in under 37 minutes or to do an extra set of repetitions in the circuit training.

If you have passed the initial fitness test which allows you to start this training schedule, there is no reason why you cannot physically complete the programme. The inhibiting factor is your mental approach to training. No-one can deny that it is not always easy to make yourself go out for a run in the rain and the dark after a particularly harassing day at work. Sometimes the thought of an hour of circuit training is enough to make you turn over and go back to sleep. This is where mental toughness plays its part. You have got to overcome the negatives and make yourself continue – and then thank yourself afterwards. There is a saying in the Regiment that is often used in training, which simply states: 'No guts, no glory.'

It is not your physical ability that will prevent you from achieving your goal (barring injury) but your mental approach. In your heart of hearts, you will know if you are making excuses to yourself as to why you cannot complete an event or start a certain training session. Obviously, you must not push yourself through injury – that is not the purpose of developing mental toughness. But you must be able to recognise when you are 'wimping out', when you are simply tiring yet still have more to give, when you are experiencing the normal discomfort of hard training as opposed to the pain of injury. In these instances, it is mental muscle – your state of mind – that will help you complete the session.

One of the unique features of The Parachute Regiment is their wicked and black sense of humour. A joke or a quip at the right time can have an amazing effect on sinking morale and the P Company staff use humour exhaustively and to great effect during training. Paras have a great knack of being able to laugh at themselves and the idiocy of a situation. As you struggle through your umpteenth hill rep, a wry smile at the lunacy of what you're doing when you could be down the pub can lift the spirits enormously.

Additionally, when preparing for P Company, the recruits have the extra bonus of camaraderie which develops in the face of overcoming a common challenge. They will encourage and help each other in events where one might be weaker than the others. They also have the staff to encourage, cajole, and harangue them when things get tough. From a motivation point of view, many find it easier to train with a partner or number of colleagues and, certainly, it can be more fun. However, never forget that ultimately, the only person you can rely on to get you through the schedule is yourself. You must believe that you can achieve your goal and go after it with determination.

Paras exhibit a pride in their Regiment and an arrogance that is infuriating to other units of the army. It makes them a lot of enemies but it also achieves results. They believe completely, they know utterly that they are the best and because of this, they are a formidable foe and unlikely to fail. Small wonder that they dominate army sporting competitions and are feared by armies around the world.

None of us likes to lose face, and the fear of failing in front of their peers and the P Company staff, whose respect they crave, is a great motivator

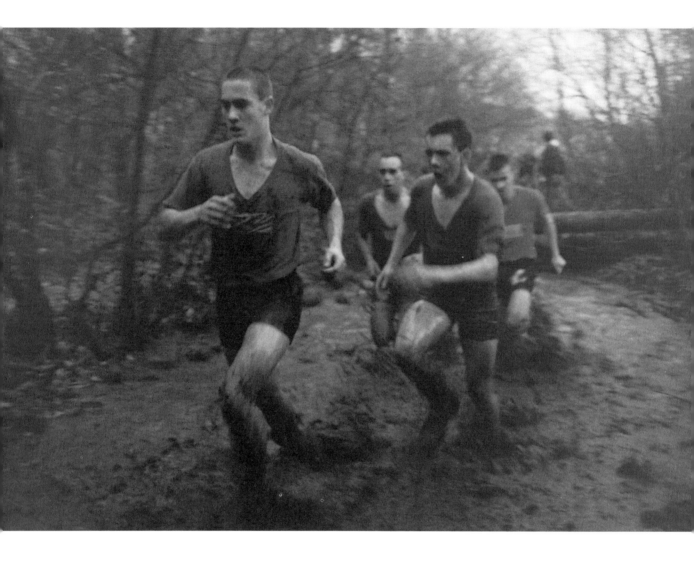

for recruits. When training alone, this element is missing but, having once told their wife, family and friends that they are going to start The Paras Ultimate Fitness Training Programme, the thought of publicly admitting that they've given up is enough to keep some demoralised souls going. One of the principles of P Company is that: 'Fear of failure must be greater than fear of the apparatus or task ahead.'

If you believe in yourself, if only to complete this training programme, then, when you are successful, it will raise your self-esteem immeasurably. This has a knock-on effect in every aspect of your life. The Regiment reports that two of the positive outcomes for the young men who pass P Company are that there is a reduction in aggression since they no longer need to prove themselves to others once they have proved to themselves that they are mentally (and physically) tough; and that once they are confident in their own fitness and strength, they are more likely to help others.

Another useful tool in the armoury of mental preparation is to use mental practice, also known as mental rehearsal or visualisation techniques. It is not commonly used in military training except perhaps when training men to fix bayonets and charge dug-in enemy trenches, but it has been known to produce good results in the coaching environment of a number of sporting bodies, particularly athletics, weightlifting and combat sports. Great exponents of mental rehearsal include Linford Christie (see the concentration on his face before any race), the late Arthur Ash, the former Wimbledon tennis champion, and the boxer Chris Eubank.

Captain Jim Wood BEM of the army physical training corps, who works in liaison with The Parachute Regiment, says:

'Mental rehearsal can be employed in a wide variety of settings in order to elicit improved performance. It can further improve self-mastery in environments that are alien to the individual and develop the mental toughness that is required of both athlete and soldier alike. Mental rehearsal of a coming event or test can provide greater self-confidence and help to control anxiety levels, so generating more positive anticipation for the desired outcome.'

To use mental rehearsal effectively, you must believe in its benefits. For some, visualising themselves completing an event or successfully going through the skills needed to overcome a challenge works well. For others, positive thoughts or internal verbalisations such as 'I know I can' are more effective. Mentally rehearsing your performance before and between trials is a good practice to get into and 'psyching yourself up' at times of low morale is also a useful ploy.

This technique is particularly useful when you fail to achieve one of your targets, as you almost certainly will. If and when this happens, don't be too hard on yourself. Rather than viewing it as a failure or unproductive, see it as a stepping stone to future success. Take a positive approach to it and see tomorrow as another day. Continuing after a set-back is the true measure of mental toughness and determination.

Unfortunately, the power of the mind is just as strong whether it is used positively or negatively. The staff of P Company see this time and time again when recruits who are physically well prepared and able to complete P Company Test Week are defeated because the test takes on insurmountable proportions in their minds. They convince themselves before the week even begins that they cannot possibly pass it and so they fail. This is incredibly frustrating for the staff who are well aware of an individual recruit's capabilities but, basically, no amount of encouragement or avowing of their ability can overcome a recruit's mental block. They will almost certainly be sent back for retraining and to try again, if they have the mental resilience to go through it all again.

So, it is essential to stay positive and, to do so, use any device available to you to improve your self-confidence and self-esteem. A good trick is to redo the initial fitness tests as you progress through the training schedule. You will be amazed by how much your performance has improved. Similarly, doing the pulse test throughout the 16-week training period is a good yardstick by which to measure your fitness progress. It can give your confidence a great boost and inspire you to greater efforts.

When training as a squad, there are always those who fall behind the pace. Psychologically, it is then extremely hard for them to make up that distance and catch up with their peers, particularly when they are not only feeling exhausted but demoralised as well. Most of the P Company staff have an imaginary line of 50 yards behind the main group and if a recruit falls behind that line, then they are unlikely to make up the ground and have failed the test.

However, there are the brave few who, against all the odds, overcome the seemingly insurmountable mental hurdle and actually catch up. They draw on great depths of determination and resilience. The ability to push ourselves that little bit harder, to give that little bit more when it feels like we've given our all is within each of us and it's simply a case of recognising the fact.

It can be taken to its extreme. Stories abound of recruits so keen to earn their red beret that they complete P Company Test Week with injuries such as fractures and shin splints. This is not to be recommended and I don't advocate training through injury.

The purpose of this chapter is not to preach or be puritanical but simply to stress the importance of a holistic approach to training. It takes mental as well as physical training to become truly fit. The Parachute Regiment recognises this fact and sets as much store by a recruit's mental approach and attitude as by his physical ability. Hopefully, it will stand you in good stead too.

Men Apart or Mere Mortals?

Most paratroopers, when pressed, will confess that there were times during training and P Company Test Week when they came close to quitting. The fact that they are wearing the red beret today is evidence that they passed through this crisis and carried on against seemingly insurmountable odds. Yet, each faced those moments of doubt. What got them through?

Why does one man find the necessary resolve while others fail? The answer is unfathomable but here is a selection of comments on personal motivation taken from a group of men who were going through the hell of P Company at the time of questioning.

Although highly personal to the individual, the answers seem to fall into a number of distinct categories.

Primarily, there is the impetus of wanting something so badly that you push yourself through almost anything:

'I had wanted to be a paratrooper since I joined the army and nothing is going to get in the way of what I want to be'

Gnr Ream

'The thought of wearing the red beret spurred me on.'

Spr Forrester

For many, fear of failure or losing face plays a very large part:

'Having to face all the wasters who would never attempt the course but would be quick enough to take the piss had I jacked kept me going.'

CFN Kerr

'I wasn't going to quit or let myself down by failing.'

Gnr Ream

'Even when my legs just wouldn't work and I fell back behind the squad by two minutes on the fourteen mile endurance march, the thought of being disgraced and put on the wagon kept me going and when I caught them up at the tea stop, it lifted me. Once I had proved to myself that I could go on, it got easier and I stayed with the squad the rest of the way.'

Spr Parker

'Even though you're knackered, I thought of my own reason for coming on the course which was to prove to myself that I could complete the hardest physical course in the army.'

Sgt Hastings

'There have been times during marches when I have been behind the squad and

thought "I'll never catch up!" But the fear of being told to get on the "Jack wagon" kept me going. I wish I had £1 for every time I've been called a "tosser".'

LCPL Hoggarth

Characterised by a feeling of team spirit, this stimulus is only applicable to those training with others:

'The comradeship on the course between students is fantastic. There's always someone to help or offer advice.'

'Motivation is the instructor four inches from my face screaming at me to get a move on, and the fact that I was f****d if I was going to get in the wagon and make his day.'

LCPL Clarke

'A lot of it is down to the staff keeping everyone together as a squad. On individual events, it's down to yourself whether you want it badly enough or not. In the team events, you want to give a little bit extra so as not to let any members of the team down.'

LCPL Boydell

For the pragmatists, the reasons are naturally practical:

'All the hard work on my beat-up (preparation course) and on the course so far was too much to go through to give up then.'

Spr Forrester

'After getting this far, it would be a waste to jack it in then.'

LCPL Boydell

'The thought of missing out on an extra £110 per month.'

LCPL Haywood

(Paras get extra pay in recognition of the additional demands placed upon them.)

Finally, for some this may be the last chance to realise a lifelong ambition and so the thought of failing is insupportable:

'This is the only time in my life I will be able to try P Company.'

Capt McColl

The reasons for finding that little bit extra vary from person to person and for some the motivation is multi-faceted. Somehow, it is strangely comforting to know that paratroopers have the same foibles, moments of weakness and self-doubt as the rest of us. What makes them, and potentially you, so special is having the courage to overcome the temptation to give up and, even in their darkest moments, finding the strength to carry on.

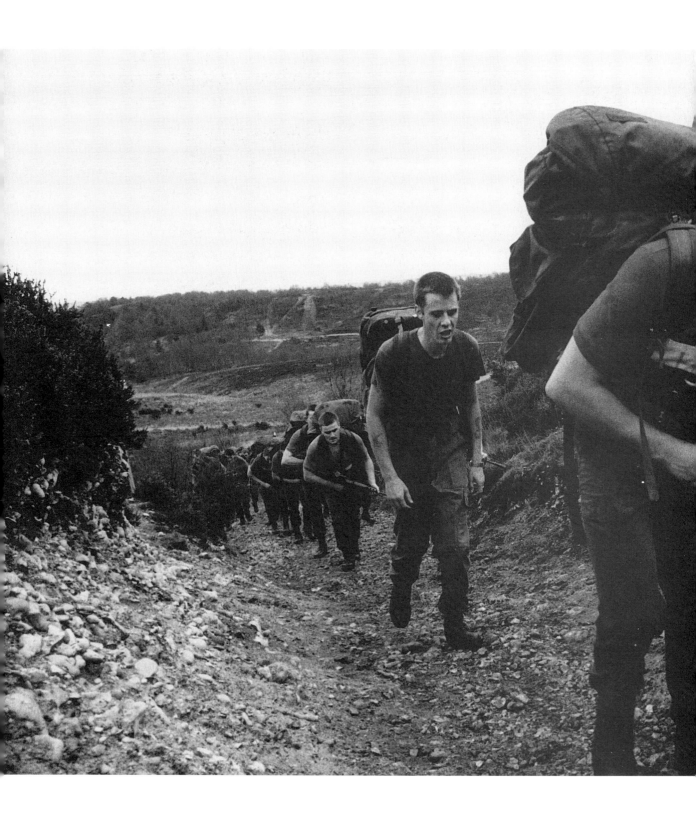

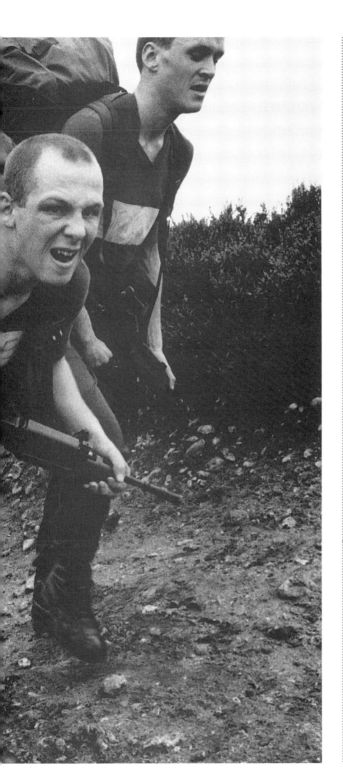

Chapter Five

Dealing With Injuries

· ·

One of the disadvantages of any intensive training programme is that there are common training injuries associated with placing the body under continued physical stress. However, by following the precautions and golden rules of training outlined in Chapter 3 Preparation, many of these niggling injuries can be avoided. Nonetheless, the Paras have years of experience of dealing with training damage. So, if you do fall prey to injury, here are a few tips on how to treat the more common afflictions.

Prevention is the best form of first aid. Make sure you are using the correct equipment, and remember that a well-made pair of running shoes is one of the most important contributions you can make in preventing injuries. Use the best you can afford, make sure they fit properly, and discard shoes if they are badly worn.

Be sensible and take the necessary rest from training when it is called for but also bear in mind that, on a bad day, anybody can feel as if they have an injury.

Blisters

Ensure that you're wearing a good, well-fitting pair of training shoes when running. Also ensure that your socks do not have seams in them as these can cause blisters.

Every Para has his own tried and tested method of preventing blisters, ranging from talcum powder and/or Vaseline on friction areas such as tops of toes, heels, etc. to wearing two pairs of socks. Unfortunately, for a Para, particularly in training, blisters are an occupational hazard.

Treatment
Received wisdom recommends cleaning the area with antiseptic lotion. Use a pin sterilised in flame, then cooled, to prick the bubble, releasing fluid.

Apply a liberal covering of antiseptic cream. Formerly, protection of the treated area required leaving the skin in place, covering with gauze, and then adhesive tape on top. When training, Paras used slippery plaster and greased the outside of the tape with soap. However, the latest recommendation to runners is to apply an elasticated stretch adhesive bandage BPC with the sticky side directly on to the blister, and to leave this in place for 10 days, thus sealing the lesion and preventing infection. By all accounts, the results are miraculous.

Sprain, Strain and Contusion

These are progressive injuries. A **sprain** is the stretching or tearing of ligament tissue. Its symptoms are discomfort and limited tenderness to the touch.

Treatment for a sprain
Treatment involved RICE:

- Rest,
- Ice,
- Compression, and
- Elevation.

See end of chapter for a fuller description. Use ice pack for approximately 20–30 mins.

A **strain** is the overstretching or tearing of a muscle or tendon. It is a moderate injury which is tender to the touch, possibly involving muscle spasm. Range of motion is painful. There is often swelling and possible discolouration.

Treatment for a strain

RICE and support. In moderate or severe cases, treat every hour or when pain is experienced. In less severe cases, treat as symptoms dictate. Continue treatment for at least 24–72 hours depending on the severity of the injury. For mild to moderate strains, gradual stretching to the point of pain is recommended.

A **contusion** is caused by impact force resulting in the bleeding of underlying tissue. Severe tearing or complete rupture of the tissue results. Symptoms are extreme tenderness to the touch, and possible loss of function. Swelling and muscle spasm are likely to be present, with discolouration and possible deformity.

Treatment for a contusion

RICE. It is also advisable to see your G.P.

Heel Bruise (stone bruise)

Often the result of unaccustomed road work, this is felt as a severe pain caused by a sudden abnormal impact to the heel area. It causes immediate disability and may develop into a chronic inflammatory condition of the periosteum (the tissue surrounding all bone surfaces).

Treatment

RICE. Apply a pad for comfort on weight bearing. To prevent this condition, wear well-cushioned training shoes with firm heel pads. Avoid road running and move to grass or a parkland venue.

Shin Splints

This is an overuse injury tending to occur in novices running on hard surfaces. Worn soles and constant running on the same side of a cambered road also contribute. Shin splints are felt as a dull ache in the lower leg region. There will be a decrease in performance due to soft tissue pain. There may be mild swelling and heat along the area of inflammation. Pain is felt on moving the foot up and down.

Treatment

At first sign of pain, rest. RICE after use. Contrast baths or compresses (warm bath for 20 mins; ice for 20 mins). When symptoms subside, return to running on soft surfaces. If symptoms persist, seek medical advice.

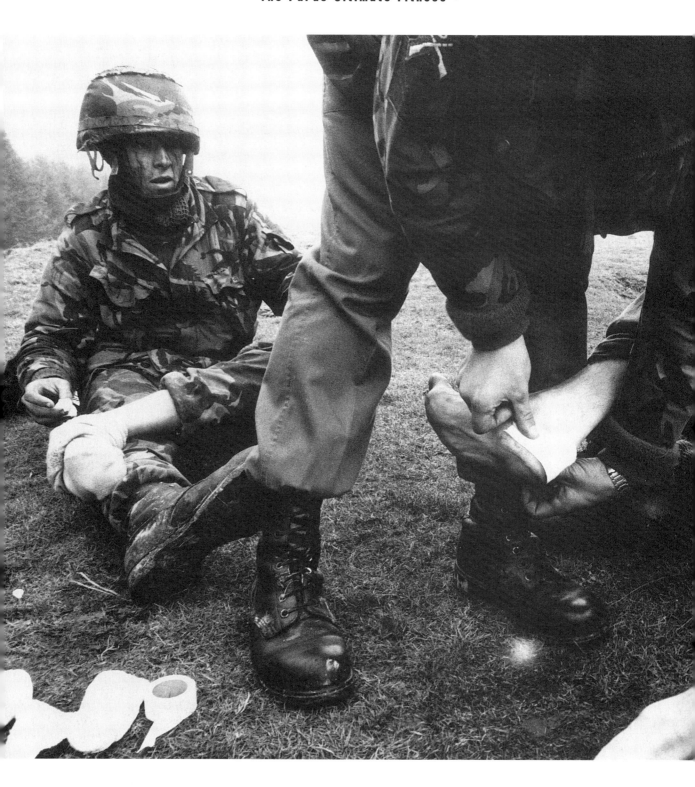

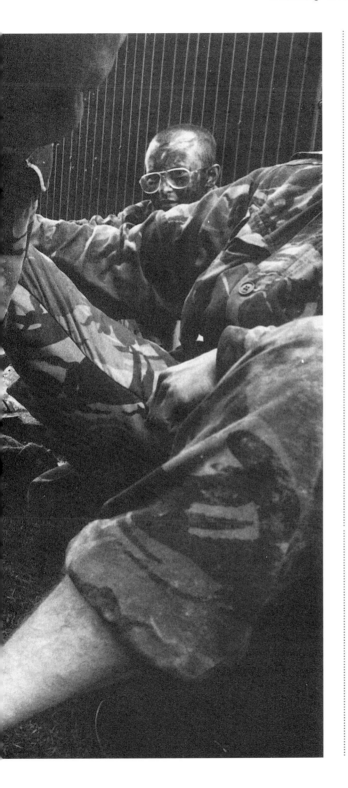

Achilles Tendon Pain (Tendinitis)

This is felt as a burning pain in the thick tendon of the calf muscle which subsides during a run and then becomes more severe afterwards. A lump may develop if the injury is not allowed to heal properly. Symptoms include stiffness in the morning; pain when rising on tiptoes; pain on running. May be caused by hill running to excess, unstable shoes, or shoes with rigid soles.

Treatment

RICE. Hot and cold compresses. Heel raise.

Sprained Ankle

Usually caused by 'turning' the foot over on rough ground. Symptoms are immediate pain followed by swelling. Over the next 10 minutes, the pain will subside and, in the case of a moderate strain, you can hobble on. In severe cases, you will not be able to put any weight on the foot.

Treatment

RICE followed by strapping with non-elastic adhesive strapping BPC. In severe cases (when you can't bear weight) go to the casualty department of the local hospital.

Runner's Knee

Distinguished by an aching soreness around or behind the kneecap.

Treatment

RICE. Once pain free, start with gentle resistance exercises on the straightened leg, progressing to bent-leg lifting.

Hamstring Strains and Pulls

Often caused by inadequate stretching before and after training. Hill reps, interval and fartlek training are also indicated.

Treatment

Rest. The dramatic pull must be treated with ICE treatment.

Athlete's foot

This is a fungus growing between the toes, and is picked up in swimming pools and communal showers. Avoid by wearing 'flip-flops' and drying feet thoroughly.

Treatment

Treat with anti-fungal powder, liquid or cream and consult your G.P. if the problem persists.

Cramp

This is an involuntary shortening of the muscle.

Treatment

Stretch the muscle and massage it firmly.

Faintness

This is a warning that all is not well.

Treatment

Sit with your head between your knees or lie down. Cool down after a long run to avoid feeling faint again once you stand up.

Stitch

A pain under the ribs when running. The cause is not known but it may be connected with blood being taken away from digestion. Avoid training soon after eating.

Treatment

None, unfortunately.

Winding

Treatment

Breathe in 'short' then breathe out 'long' to relax the muscles.

Your basic sports injury kit

Collect together these basic items of first aid and you'll be able to treat any minor ailments or injuries you may pick up during training.

Essentials

- Box of different-sized dressing plasters.
- 4x4in sterile gauze pads (a clean handkerchief will do at a push).
- 2in gauze bandages.
- 1in and 3in elastic bandages.
- 3in non-elastic strapping.
- Icepack (plastic bags of ice or a packet of frozen peas will do).
- Scissors.

Optional

- Safety pins.
- Nail clippers.
- Needle.
- Cotton wool.
- Antiseptic fluid.
- Petroleum jelly.
- Elastic knee/ankle/elbow support.
- Sling.
- Painkiller (aspirin or paracetamol).
- Foot powder.
- Strapping tape.

RICE

Rest followed by ICE is the simplest yet most efficient remedy for many injuries. The combination of Ice, Compression and Elevation helps to reduce swelling and restrict the spread of bruising, both of which can slow down the healing process.

As soon as possible after injury, if called for, apply ice and bandaging and raise the injured part. The first 6 hours are the most important in which to rest the injury.

Ice

Apply an icepack (or cold water if ice is not available) to the injured area for 5 minutes every hour, if possible over 48 hours, to reduce the bleeding from torn blood vessels.

Compression

Bandage the injured area firmly (not so tightly that it is uncomfortable) in order to contain the swelling.

Elevation

Allow blood to return to the heart by raising the injured area, thus reducing the pressure on the injured area.

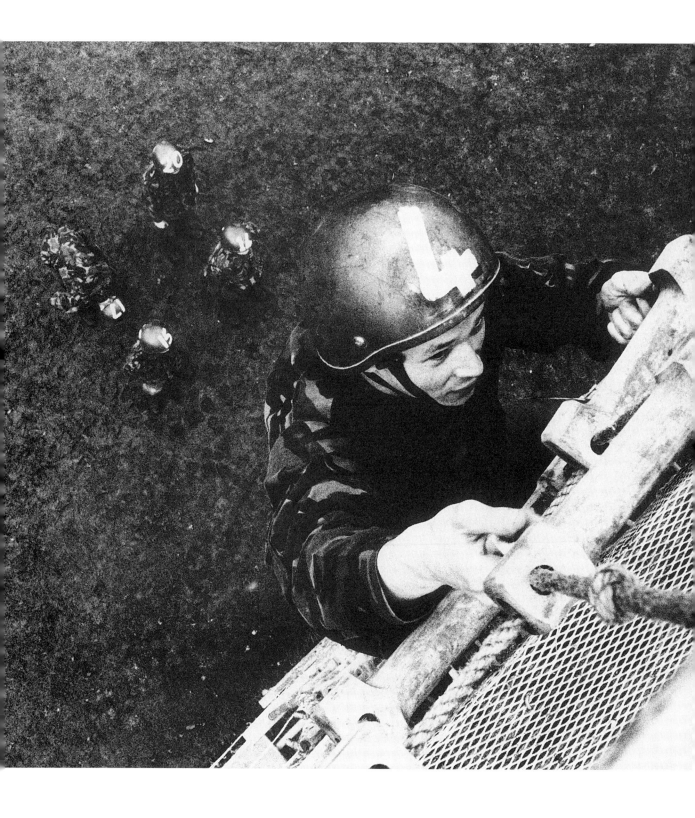

Chapter Six

Nutrition for Training

• •

It is now widely recognised that what you eat can positively or adversely affect your health. As an extension of this principle, if you tailor your diet appropriately during your training period, it has been shown that you can get better results. In fact, when they are on exercise, members of The Parachute Regiment are allocated more rations with a higher calorific value than those issued to other units of the British Army in recognition of the high physical demands placed on them.

The following is a brief explanation of the theory behind nutrition for training, plus advice on the kinds of foods you should be consuming during your 16-week training.

Carbohydrate

Carbohydrate is the most important fuel for working muscles and should make up the bulk of your diet when training. Foods rich in carbohydrates include:

- pasta,
- wholemeal bread,
- rice,
- potatoes,
- breakfast cereals,
- fruit, and
- pulses.

Make sure you get a good balance of these foods in your diet. Unfortunately, your body's stores of carbohydrate (glycogen) are fairly limited and you must keep replacing the carbohydrates as you use them. If you don't, you will start to feel tired and find it hard to complete your training session. You need to eat within the first two hours after each training session. If you cannot have a meal during this time, you will have to rely on carbohydrate-rich snack foods such as:

- bananas,
- dried fruit,
- cereal bars,
- jam sandwiches,
- malt loaf,
- scones,
- currant buns, and
- chocolate bars or drinks.

Fat

In our highly processed western diet, there is plenty of opportunity for us to take in fat in our diet. There is certainly no need actively to increase your fat intake when training. The body's fat stores are plentiful, even in the leanest athlete.

Protein

It is not protein itself that your body needs but a sufficient quantity of the amino acids which proteins yield when broken down in the gut. Amino acids are required primarily to manufacture the structural components of tissues such as muscle. Protein deficiency in an athlete is rare and, in general, we consume too much. There is little evidence to suggest you need to

increase your protein intake, even during heavy training.

Fluids

Keep up your fluid intake throughout training. You must replace fluids lost in sweat, otherwise your body becomes dehydrated and less efficient. Also drink plenty of fluids after training. If you get bored with water, vary your fluid intake to include soft drinks, isotonic drinks and even hot drinks. A good guide to whether you are drinking enough fluids is your urine, which should be a pale straw colour and abundant.

Alcohol is a diuretic. A pint of beer produces more than a pint of urine, and spirits are even worse. Try to avoid their dehydrating effects when training seriously.

Supplements

The British Association of Sport and Medicine advises that vitamin and mineral supplements are not essential provided you have a mixed diet with plenty of fresh fruit and vegetables or fruit juice. Large doses of vitamins and mineral supplements do not boost performance. Additional salt is rarely necessary unless training in very hot weather.

When training hard, a man should consume an average energy intake of between 2,900 and 3,350 kcals per day and 72–84g of protein. For an active woman, the energy intake should be around 2,500 kcals and about 62g of protein.

Carbohydrates should account for 50–55% of the energy intake with fats (30–35%) and proteins (10–12%) making up the remainder of the diet.

Top Tips for a basic training diet

- You must consume sufficient energy in the form of carbohydrates to maintain the energy stores within the muscles (glycogen).
- Start the refuelling process as soon as you can after you finish training. The muscles' capacity to refuel is at its greatest during the first hour after training.
- Fit your eating around training. If you miss breakfast to train, have a high-carbohydrate mid-morning snack (muesli, banana sandwich etc). If you train in the evening, eat something at around 3–4pm and

have your main meal after training.

- Eat smaller but more frequent meals, and several snacks as your appetite increases.
- Use your rest days to eat sensibly and make up for any hurried meals eaten during training.
- Place the emphasis on starchy rather then sugary foods when attempting to increase your carbohydrate intake.
- Try to cut down on sugary foods, pies, pastries, and fried foods.

Healthy Living

About 20 years ago, a set of recommendations for healthy eating was published in the USA. Since then, most western countries have promoted similar goals. The main points are:

- ✓ Control energy intake (i.e. calories).
- ✓ Eat less fat, particularly saturated fat.
- ✓ Eat more starchy foods rich in fibre.
- ✓ Eat less refined and processed sugar.
- ✓ Eat less salt.
- ✓ Drink less alcohol.

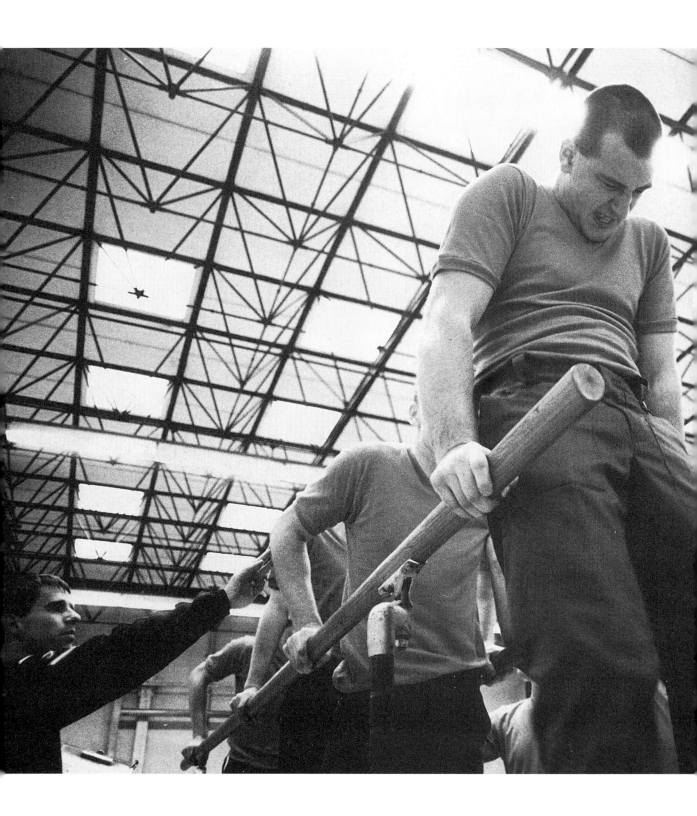

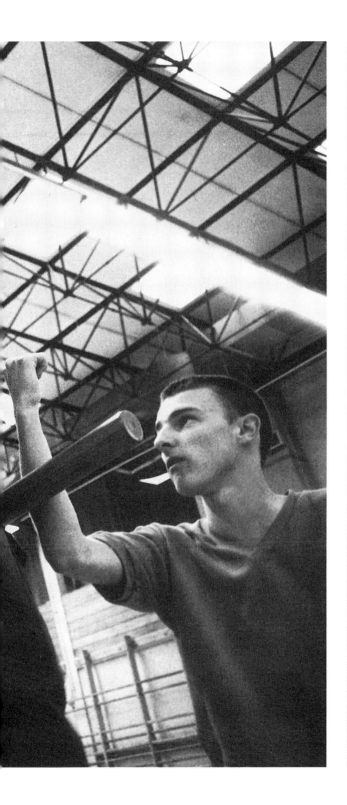

Chapter Seven

The Paras Ultimate Fitness Training Programme

• •

Time allowed for each training session include a warm-up and cool-down period of a minimum of 10 minutes each. Refer to Chapter 3, pages 35 – 46 for details of the warm-up and cool-down exercises.

Space your training sessions sensibly. Never attempt to cram the sessions into a weekend, for example. It is imperative that you take adequate rest between training sessions and that you only attempt one training session per day.

It is possible to substitute some of the training sessions of The Paras Ultimate Fitness Training Programme with other activities. You will find a comparison of activities and their physiological benefits in Chapter 8, Maintaining Fitness. Various activities are listed by category, and you should obviously select an alternative from the relevant category. However, do not forget the warm-up, cool-down and stretching/flexibility aspects in addition to the sport itself. Moreover, this should be a rarity rather than a regular occurrence otherwise you will find that you keep avoiding the harder training sessions or replacing those elements of the programme you don't enjoy with a recreational sport you do. Don't give in to temptation.

Irrespective of how well you did on the fitness testing section, I recommend that you follow the programme in its entirety. Obviously, if you did well, you will find the first few weeks very easy but it is a wise precaution.

Below, you will find a key to the areas of the body worked by or benefitting from specific exercises or activities:

CR   Cardio-respiratory
LME Local muscular endurance
LL   Lower Limb
UL   Upper Limb
A   Abdominal
L   Lumbar
F   Flexibility
S   Strength

In addition, swimming works the upper and lower limbs and promotes cardio-respiratory performance and local muscular endurance. Running reaps the same benefits with the exception of the upper limbs.

The Paras incorporate a great deal of running in their training schedule for the reasons already outlined in Chapter 1. To keep the training varied, different styles of running are used including fartlek, speed reps, hill reps and interval training. For a definition of these forms of training, see p116 at the end of this chapter.

Don't forget to reconnoitre routes for runs well in advance and to prepare any necessary equipment for a weekly programme in good time.

I have included for your interest a key to the recruits' dress code for the following training sessions:

B   Boots

B&B   Boots and bergen

B&H   Boots and helmet

You will also find an indication of the sort of weights they would be carrying in their bergens (rucksacks) in brackets next to the length of the run. This is purely for information and it is not recommended that you emulate this unless you are hell-bent on training with weight. However, it does affect the time allowed for certain events; where weights are included, the times have not been adjusted.

All that is left for me to say is, be 'Ready For Anything' and best of luck.

REMEMBER

1. Warm up and cool down thoroughly during every session (timings allow for a minimum of 10 mins warm-up and cool-down and, for more demanding sessions, 15 mins respectively).

2. Only one session per day and take the necessary rest periods.

3. Carrying weight is not recommended. It is simply optional.

4. Repeat a week if you feel it is necessary to stay at a certain level. Avoid moving the sessions around within the week if possible. Once you start adjusting the programme, mentally it is easier to start dropping sessions altogether.

5. However enthusiastic, do not exceed the number of weekly sessions. Overtraining can lead to injury.

PHASE 1

This closely approximates the first 5 weeks of physical training that all army recruits can expect to follow when they arrive at Lichfield. The aim is to convert 'fat civvies' into 'lean, mean fighting machines'.

Week 1

SESSION 1 (1 HOUR)

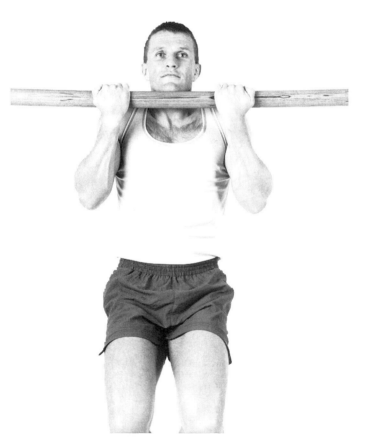

1. 10 heaves (LME, UL)

During the 16-week schedule vary the method using:

• under-grasp;

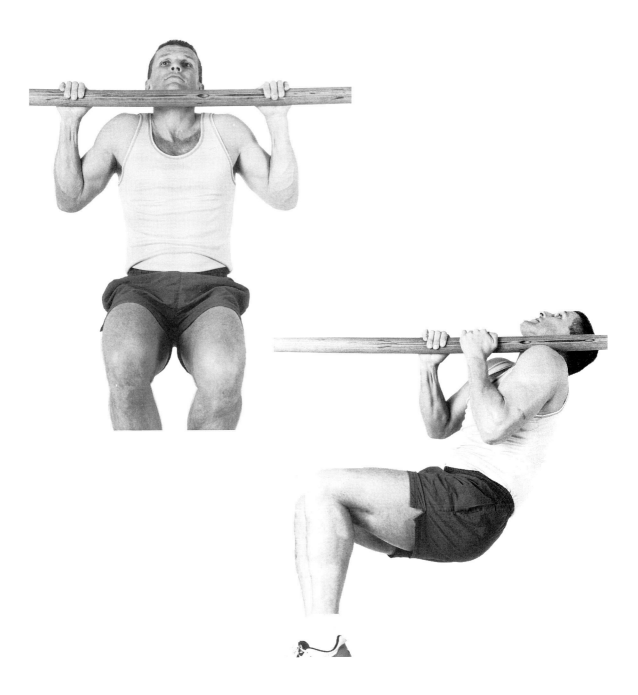

- over-grasp;
- alternate-grasp.

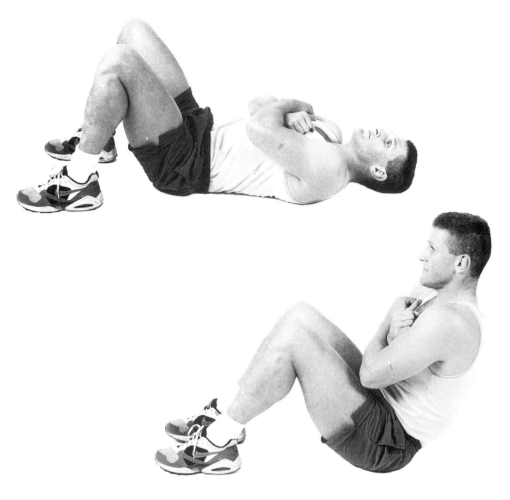

2. Abdominal exercises: 60 reps (LME)

Sit-ups:

- Lie on your back with your hands placed across your chest, knees bent, feet hip-width apart and flat on the floor. (If you have difficulties, hook your feet under a chair or bar.)
- Raise your upper body into a sitting position.
- Return to the starting position and repeat.

3. 1.5-mile (2.4km) run

To be completed in under 10 mins 30 secs.

SESSION 2 (1 HOUR)

Gym exercises (CR + LME)

3 sets of 20 reps i.e. repeat each exercise 20 times, pass to next exercise and repeat 20 times, etc. When all the exercises in the circuit are complete, return to the first exercise and repeat the whole procedure twice i.e. 3 x 20 reps.

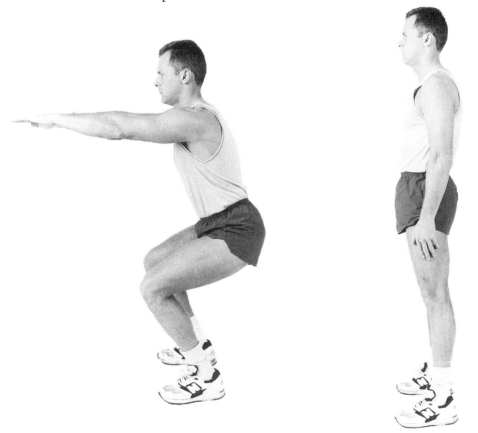

Squats (LL):

• From standing position, squat to sitting position (arms raised).

• Return to standing position and raise up onto toes. Repeat.

Sit-ups (A):

See Week 1, Session 1.

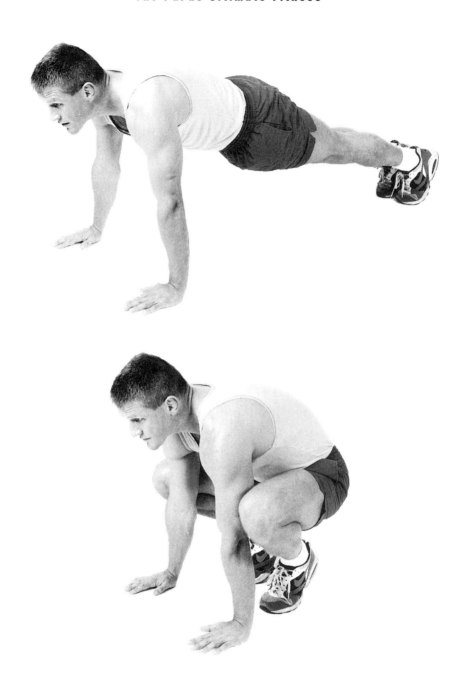

Squat Thrusts (LL):

- From squat position (knees touching elbows), thrust legs back straight.
- Jump both legs back to the starting position. Repeat.

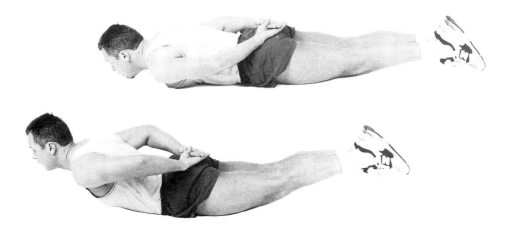

Dorsal Raises (L + F):

- Lie flat on the floor, face down and with hands clasped behind your back.
- Keeping your legs straight, raise your head and chest from the floor.
- Lower and repeat.

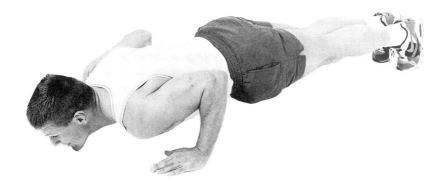

Press-ups (UL):

- Start face down, hands shoulder-width apart, legs and body straight, your head in line with your body.
- Lower your body (keeping your back straight) so that chest touches lightly on the floor.
- Push back up so arms are straightened to the original position.
- Repeat.

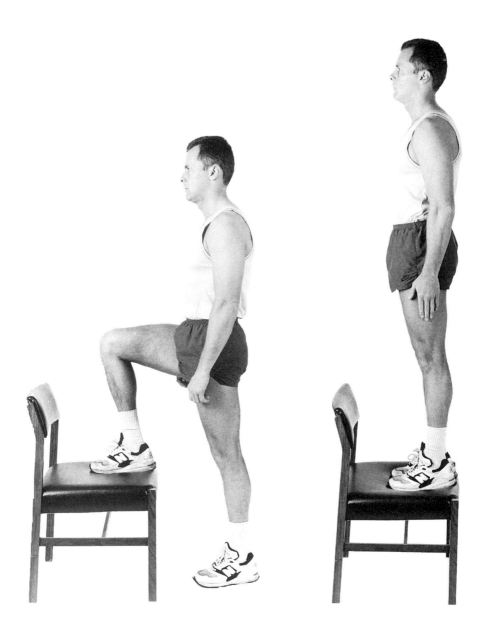

Step-Ups:

30 steps each leg (LL):

- Place one foot on chair (or step of stairs).
- Step up onto chair with legs fully extended.
- Step down leaving same foot in contact with chair.

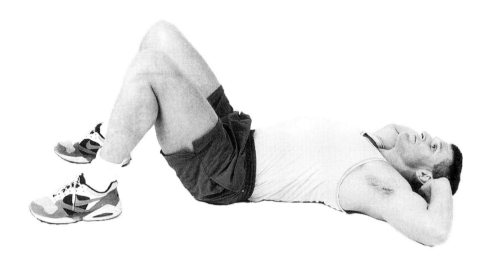

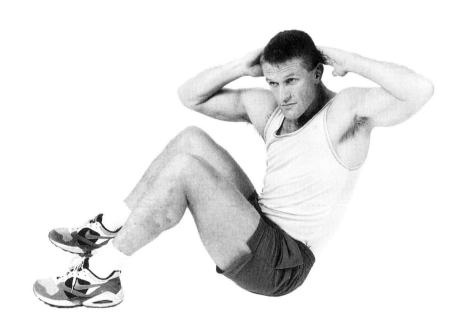

Twist Sit-ups (A + F):

- Lying on your back, hands clasped behind head, knees bent.
- Sit up and twist upper body to touch elbow on opposite knee.
- Alternate left and right.

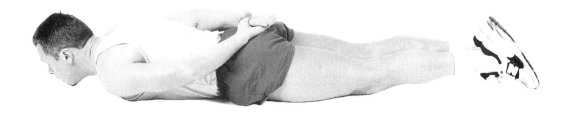

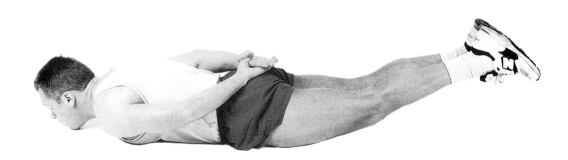

Leg Lifts (L + F):

- Lie face down with hands clasped behind your back.
- Lift both legs together from the floor and lower back to floor.
- Repeat.

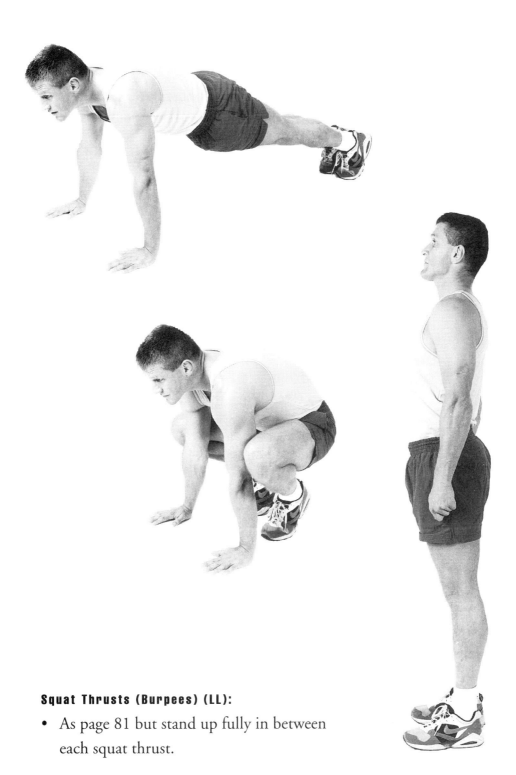

Squat Thrusts (Burpees) (LL):

- As page 81 but stand up fully in between each squat thrust.

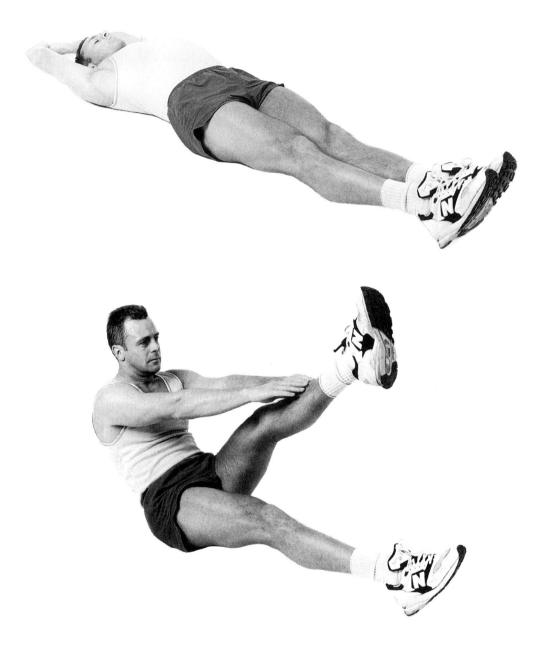

Alternative V Sits (A + F):

- Lie on back with legs straight and arms extended above head.
- Lifting one leg straight, sit up and reach towards ankle of rising leg.
- Alternate leg raising.

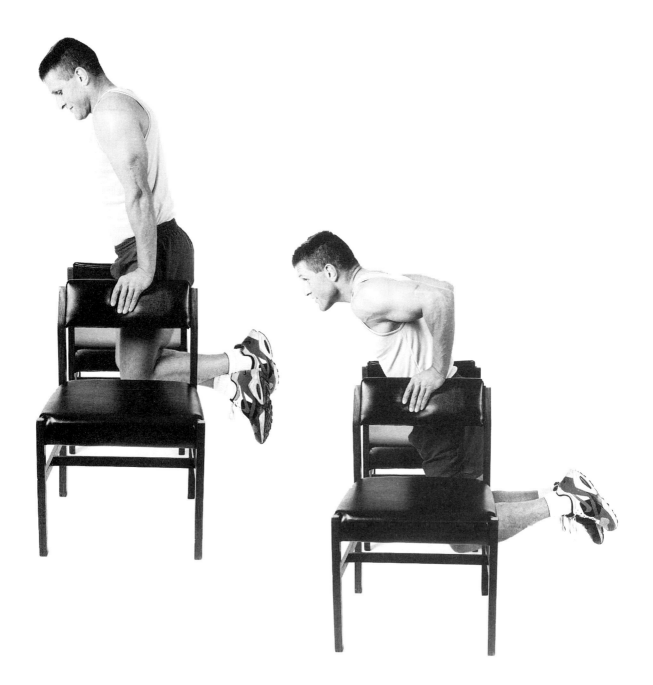

Dips (UL):

- Hands resting on the back of two chairs, legs bent, lower towards floor.
- Push back until arms fully extended.

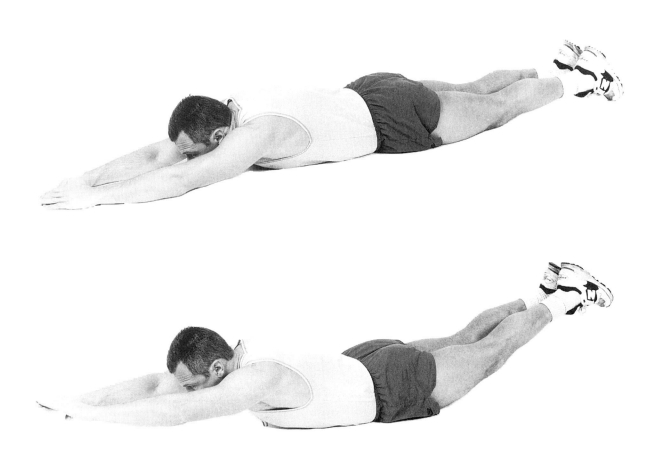

Advanced Dorsal (L + F):

• Lie on your front, arms out straight by head.

• Raise arms, chest and legs from the floor and lower.

SESSION 3 (1–1 HOUR 30 MINS)

5-mile (8km) run

To be completed at your own pace.

SESSION 4 (1 HOUR)

5-mile run

Aim for a pace of c. 8 mins/mile.

Week 2

SESSION 1 (1 HOUR)

5-mile run

To be completed at c. 8 mins/mile pace.

SESSION 2 (1 HOUR)

Swimming

- Jump in.
- Tread water for 2 mins (1 min using arms and legs, 1 min just legs).
- Swim 100m any stroke, no time limit (not allowed to touch sides or bottom of pool).
- Climb out at deep end without using steps.

SESSION 3 (1 HOUR)

5-mile run

At 8 mins/mile pace.

SESSION 4 (1 HOUR)

Running Circuit

3 sets of 20 reps with a 20–50m run between each set i.e. 20 press-ups, run, 20 sit-ups, run etc.

- Press-ups.
- Sit-ups.
- Step-ups.
- Dips.

SESSION 5 (1 HOUR 30 MINS)

1. 5-mile run

   At 8 mins/mile pace.

2. Running Circuit

   Finish with 1 set of 50 reps of the above running circuit.

Week 3

SESSION 1 (1 HOUR)

Interval Training

This subjects the body to short, regular, repeated bouts of work interspersed with rest periods. The work requires maximum effort e.g. sprinting, swimming, cycling. Distances can vary between 50m to 200m for these maximum efforts and the pulse rate should rise to a maximum of 85% of MHR (see page 30). Intervals between maximum efforts should be long enough to allow the heart rate to drop halfway to the resting pulse rate.

The aim is to progress to a total distance at maximum effort (excluding rest periods) of:

- running – 1.5-mile/2.5km;
- swimming – 1-mile/1.5km;
- cycling – at least 2-miles/3km.

Note: if you are training with a colleague or with a group of friends, a crude form of interval training that is good fun is to use relays, lifting and carrying exercises. These include such activities as leap frog, under-and-over leap-frog, hopping over the others' legs, circle running, ball passing, relay racing, pack-a-back, carrying a man in threes etc.

SESSION 2 (1 HOUR 15 MINS) (B)
3-mile (4.8km) run/walk/run
At 15 min/mile pace.

SESSION 3 (1 HOUR)
Leisure activity
Golf, soccer, swimming etc.

SESSION 4
(1 HOUR 30 MINS – 2 HOURS)
1. 5-mile run
   At 7 mins 45 secs/mile pace.
2. Running circuit

4 sets of 20 reps (see week 2, Session 4).

SESSION 5 (1 HOUR)
Leisure activity of your choice.

Week 4
SESSION 1 (C. 1 HOUR)
5-mile run
At 7 mins 45 secs/mile pace.

SESSION 2
(1 HOUR 45 MINS) (B&B)
5-mile run (+ 20lbs weight)
To be completed in under 1 hour 15 mins.

SESSION 3 (1 HOUR) (B&H)
At this stage of the training, the recruits would be introduced to the assault course. For the purposes of this schedule, we'll substitute a gym session (see Week 1, Session 2).

SESSION 4 (2 HOURS)
Cycling, swimming or a sporting activity.

Week 5
SESSION 1 (1 HOUR)
1. 10 heaves
2. 75 sit-ups in under 4 mins
3. 1.5-mile run in 10 mins

SESSION 2 (1 HOUR)

During this session, the recruits would experience the trainasium for the first time. This is to test the ability to overcome fear while exercising.

As a substitute, we recommend something that will test your personal ability to overcome a particular fear. For example, swimming three lengths, immediately followed by a jump off the high board. (Do not attempt any activity that could cause injury.) Overcoming a fear of handling spiders is equally 'bottle' testing.

SESSION 3

(1 HOUR 30 MINS) (B&H)

5-mile march (+ 15 lbs + 9lbs weapon) At 13 mins/mile pace.

SESSION 4

(1 HOUR – 1 HOUR 20 MINS)

1. 10–30 mins cross-country run.
2. Immediately followed by continuous hill running. Up at a medium pace, down at a recovery pace, for 30 mins. Hill lengths should be 50–100m.
3. 20 mins cool-down run.

REMEMBER

1. Warm up and cool down thoroughly during every session (timings allow for a minimum of 10 mins warm-up and cool-down and, for more demanding sessions, 15 mins respectively).
2. Only one session per day and take the necessary rest periods.
3. Carrying weight is not recommended. It is simply optional.
4. Repeat a week if you feel it is necessary to stay at a certain level. Avoid moving the sessions around within the week if possible. Once you start adjusting the programme, mentally it is easier to start dropping sessions altogether.
5. However enthusiastic, do not exceed the number of weekly sessions. Overtraining can lead to injury.

PHASE 2

By now, the recruits have passed the first set of tests and they are beginning to resemble professional soldiers. At this point, grooming for the harsher physical demands of The Parachute Regiment begins.

Week 6

SESSION 1

(1 HOUR 30 MINS) (B&B)

5-mile run (+ 15 lbs + 9lbs weapon)

At 13 mins/mile pace.

SESSION 2 (2 HOURS) (B&B)

6-mile (9.6km) run (+ 15lbs + 9lbs weapon)

To be completed in 90 mins.

SESSION 3

(1 HOUR 30 MINS – 2 HOURS)

1. 5-mile run over hilly course
    At 7 mins 30 secs pace.
2. Running Circuit
    Finish with 2 sets of 20 reps of the running circuit
    (see Week 2, Session 4).

SESSION 4 (1 HOUR)

At this point, recruits are taught unarmed combat. Good equivalents are:

1. Skipping (LL + UL)
    A length of washing line will do if you don't have a skipping rope.
2. Shadow boxing (LL)
    Or controlled Karate-style chops and kicks at imaginary opponent.
3. Upper body exercises (UL)
    Dips, press-ups, dorsals, squat thrusts, wide arm press-ups etc.

Similarly to circuit training, spend 5 mins skipping before moving on to shadow boxing for 5 mins, and then upper body exercises for 5 mins. Repeat sequence again spending 10 mins on all three groups of activities.

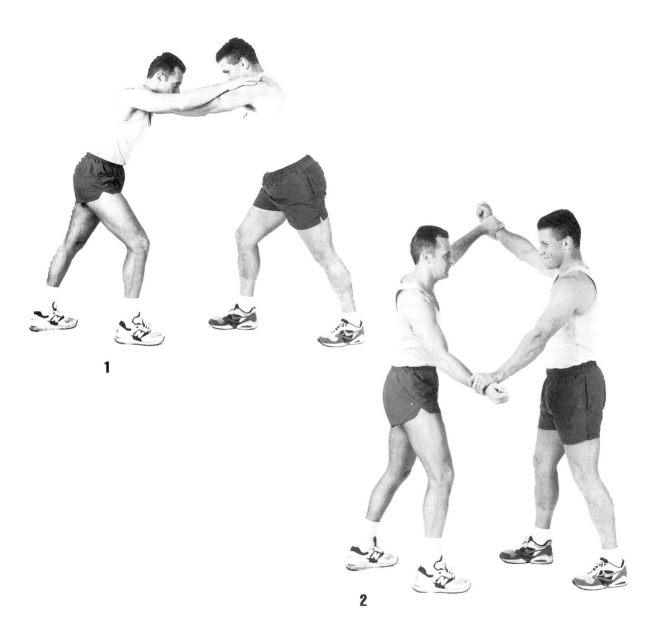

1

2

Note: if training with a partner, this is an ideal opportunity for resistance-type exercises:

1. Pushing contest with arms on each other's shoulders (LL)
2. Balance wrestling while grasping each other's wrists (UL)

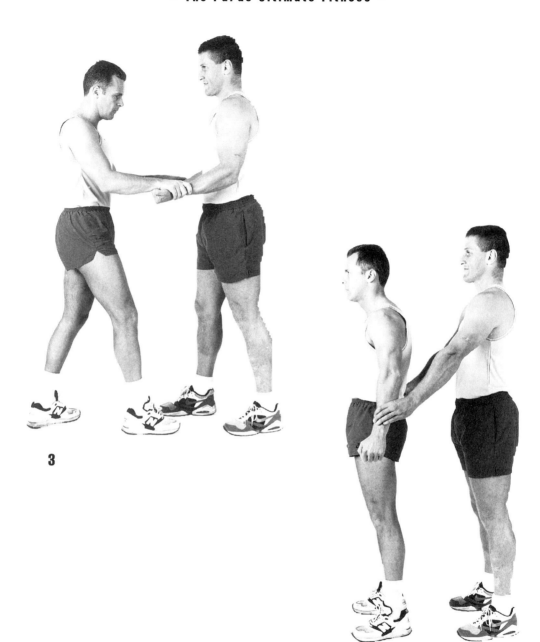

3

4

3. Resistance Curling (UL)
4. Arms raising and lowering against partner's resistance (UL)

Week 7 (recovery week)

SESSION 1
(C. 1 HOUR 30 MINS) (B&B)

6-mile run (+ 20lbs + 9lb weapon)

At 13 mins/mile pace.

SESSION 2 (2 HOURS)

1. 5-mile run incorporating hill reps
    (see Week 5, Session 4)

    At 7 mins 15 secs/mile pace.

2. Running Circuit

    Finish with running circuit of 5 sets
    of 20 reps.

Week 8

SESSION 1 (UNDER 1 HOUR)

4-mile (6.4kms) run

At 7 mins/mile pace.

SESSION 2 (2 HOURS) (B&B)

7-mile (11.2kms) march (+ 25lbs + 9lbs
weapon)

Over hilly course at 13 mins/mile pace.

SESSION 3
(1 HOUR 15 MINS) (B&H)

Recruits must complete three laps of
the assault course in under 11 mins at
this stage of the training. An equivalent
for our purposes is:

Fartlek training

45-minute session (see end of chapter
for definition).

SESSION 4 (2 HOURS)

1. Gym exercises

   See Week 1, Session 2. 3 sets of 20 reps.

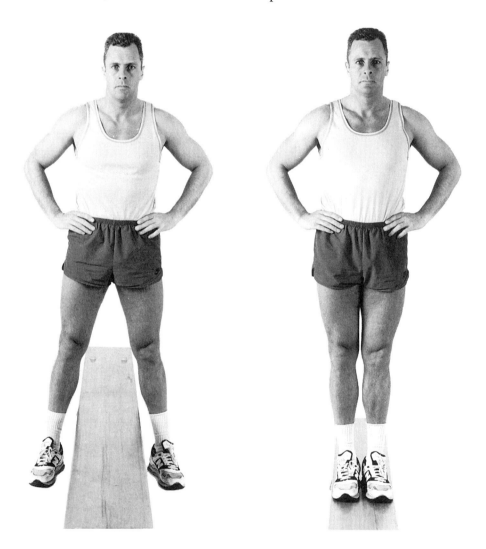

2. Plyometrics (bounding exercises)

   Running on the spot for 2 mins.

   10 reps of the following:

   Astride jumps on and off a bench or sturdy box.

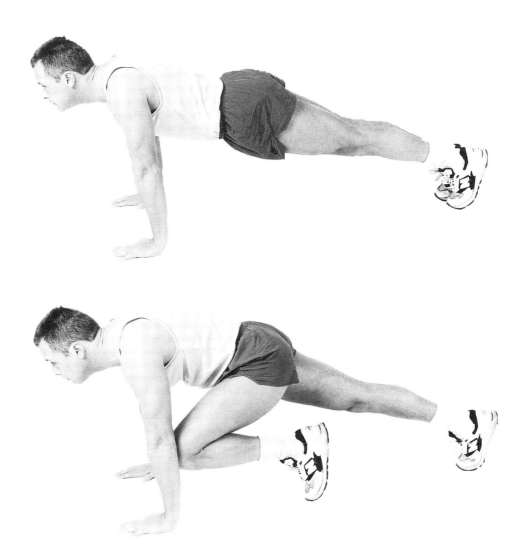

Alternate Squat Thrusts:

- Drop into press-up position.
- Bring one leg forward to chest.
- Bounce back to original position while simultaneously bringing other leg forward.

Burpees:

See Week 1, Session 2.

Tuck Jumps

- Stand with feet hip-width apart, knees slightly bent.
- Jump as high as you can, drawing the knees towards the chest (do not bring chest down to knees). Repeat.

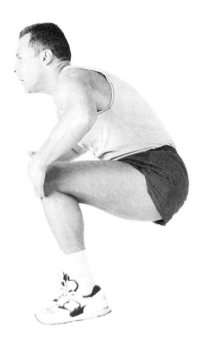

SESSION 5

(2 HOURS 15 MINS) (B&B)

1. 8-mile (12.8kms) march (+ 25lbs + 9lbs weapon)

   In 1 hour 45 mins.

2. Plyometric exercises

   See Week 8, Session 4. 10 reps each of the following:

   Running on the spot (5 mins)

   Alternate Squat Thrusts.

   Burpees.

   Tuck jumps.

Week 9

SESSION 1 (1 HOUR)

5-mile run

At 7 mins/mile pace.

SESSION 2 (1 HOUR)

Leisure activity

Cycling, swimming, squash, etc.

SESSION 3 (1 HOUR)

Circuit Training

See Week 1, Session 2.

Week 10

SESSION 1 (30–40 MINS)

1.5-mile run

In under 9 mins 30 secs.

SESSION 2 (3 HOURS) (B&B)

10-mile (16km) run (+ 25lbs + 9lbs weapon)

In 2 hours 15 mins.

SESSION 3 (45 MINS)

1. 10 heaves.

2. 90 sits-ups

   To be completed in 5 mins.

3. 1.5-mile run

   In 9 mins 30 secs.

PHASE 3

You have now surpassed the fitness goal of regular army recruits. However, this is simply the starting point of advance training for Parachute Regiment candidates.

The recruits will now be groomed by the P Company staff at Catterick for the P Company Test Week in six weeks' time. Things are intensifying: runs are getting longer; the carrying of weighted bergens and weapons is being introduced; and mental toughness is beginning to play its part.

During this phase, recruits are given an opportunity to experience and practise the skills for the assault course, trainasium, steeple chase, stretcher race and log race. These sessions are all supplementary to the training programme.

REMEMBER

1. Warm up and cool down thoroughly during every session (timings allow for a minimum of 10 mins warm-up and cool-down and, for more demanding sessions, 15 mins respectively).

2. Only one session per day and take the necessary rest periods.

3. Carrying weight is not recommended. It is simply optional.

4. Repeat a week if you feel it is necessary to stay at a certain level. Avoid moving the sessions around within the week if possible. Once you start adjusting the programme, mentally it is easier to start dropping sessions altogether.

5. However enthusiastic, do not exceed the number of weekly sessions. Overtraining can lead to injury.

Week 11

SESSION 1 (1 HOUR)

1. 1.5-miles.
   In 9 mins 30 secs.

2. 20–30 mins of
   flexibility exercises
   for legs.

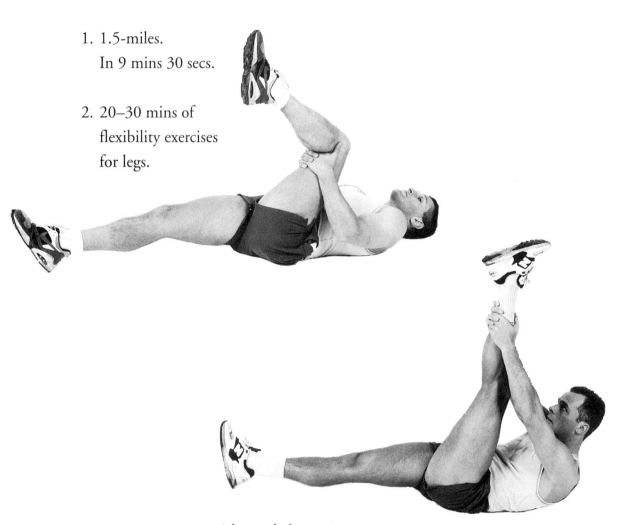

Advanced alternative

Hamstring Stretching:

- Lie flat on your back, legs straight.
- Pull one leg towards chest until stretch is felt in hamstring.
- Alternate legs.
- *Advanced alternative*: raise leg straight and pull towards head.

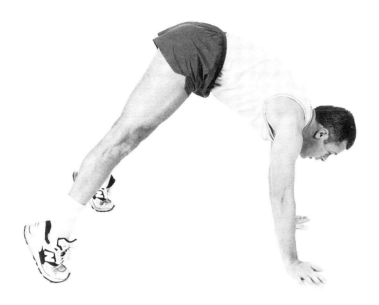

Calf Stretching:

- Bend forward until hands are flat on ground.
- Turn hands outwards.
- Walk legs back, keeping on toes until in an arched position.
- Return to starting position.

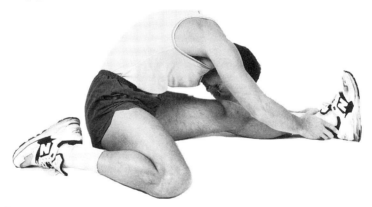

Hurdler's stretch:

- Sit with both legs straight in front of you.
- Bend one leg behind.
- Lean forward and grasp the ankle or foot of extended leg.
- Repeat on other side.

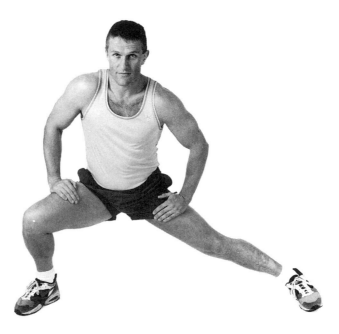

Adductor Stretch:

- Stand with legs well apart.
- Place weight over one leg and bend that leg into a squat, keeping the other leg straight.
- Repeat on other side.

SESSION 2

(2 HOURS 15 MINS) (B&B)

8-mile run (+ 30lbs + 9lbs weapon)
In 1 hour 50 mins.

SESSION 3

(2 HOURS 30 MINS) (B&B)

7-mile run with hill reps (+ 30lbs + 9lbs weapon)
See Week 5, Session 4. To be completed in 2 hours.

SESSION 4

(1 HOUR 30 MINS)

Leisure activities and sports of your choice. Choose from the list of comparable activities on pages 124–5.

Week 12

SESSION 1

(2 HOURS 30 MINS) (B&B)

10-mile run (+ 30lbs + 9lbs weapon)

In 2 hours over rough terrain.

SESSION 2 (1 HOUR)

4-mile run

Over hilly course at 8 mins/mile pace.

SESSION 3 (1 HOURS 20 MINS)

6-mile run

Over hilly course at 8 mins/mile pace.

SESSION 4 (1 HOUR 30 MINS)

Weight training and aerobic exercise

20 reps with 2–3 mins rest between exercises.

Without apparatus

See Week 1, Session 2. Press-ups:

- 10 x normal stance.
- 10 x arms narrow stance.
- 10 x arms wide stance.
- 10 x on finger tips.
- 10 x press-ups with clap.

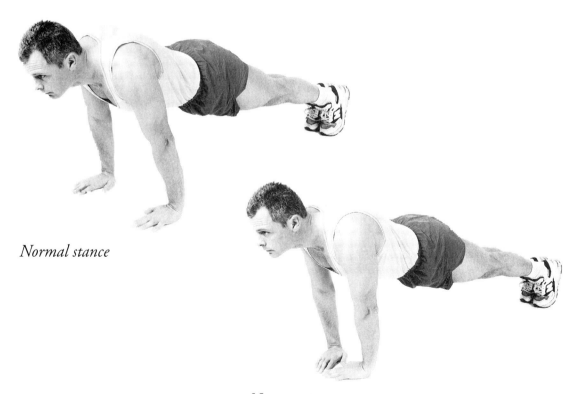

Normal stance

Narrow stance

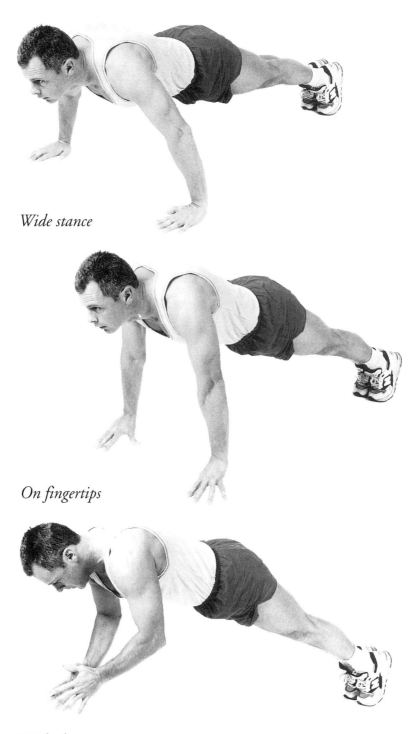

Wide stance

On fingertips

With clap

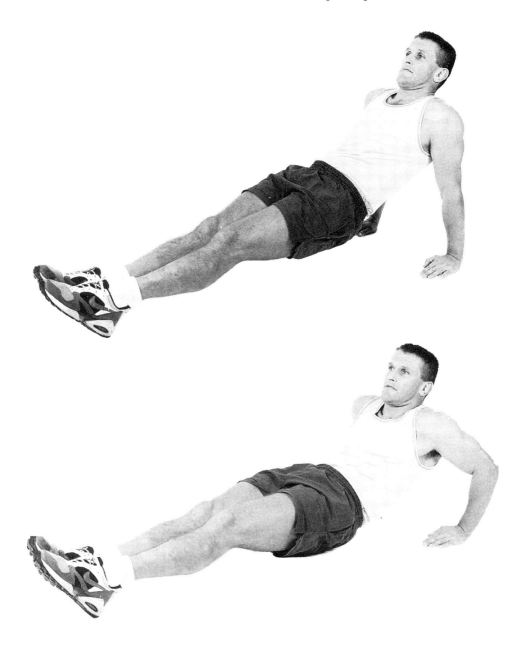

Tricep Dips:

- Lie on back.
- Raise yourself up on your arms with arms straight.
- Bend arms to lower your body with legs straight.
- Straighten arms and return to start position.

Sit-ups:

Dorsals

Astride jumps

Alternate Squat Thrusts

Burpees

Heaves

Dips

See Week 1, Session 2

With Weights

If you have no access to a supervised weights room, use a broom handle with buckets of sand tied on as improvisation at home. Keep weight to a minimum.

When training with weights, always ask a friend to act as a 'stand-in' in case you have to drop the weight. If training alone, never go beyond your comfortable limit.

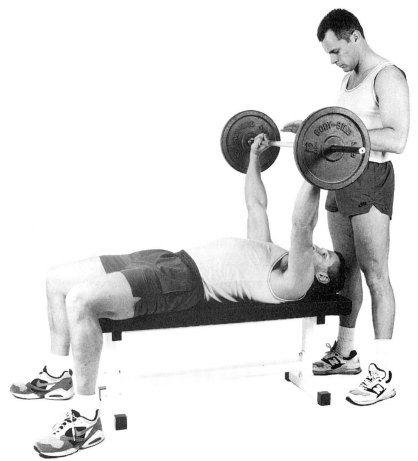

Bench press (LME + S)

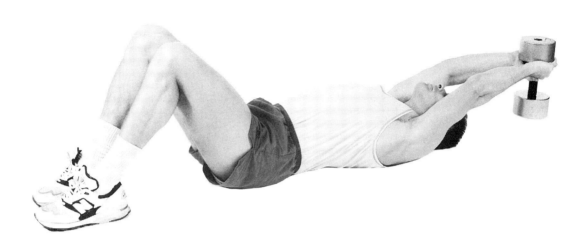

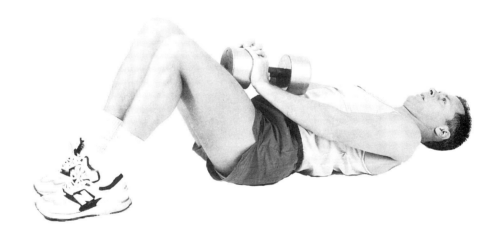

Straight arm pullovers (UL + F + S)

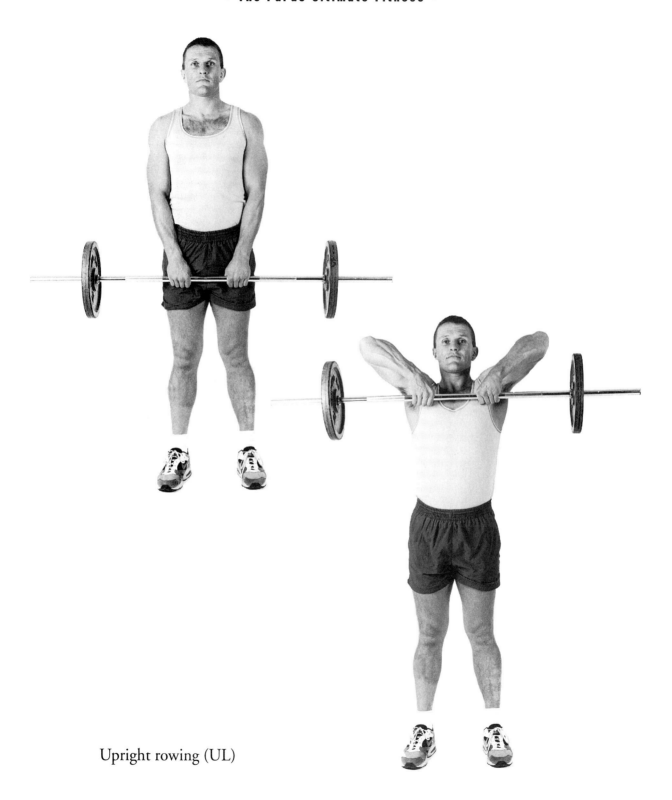

Upright rowing (UL)

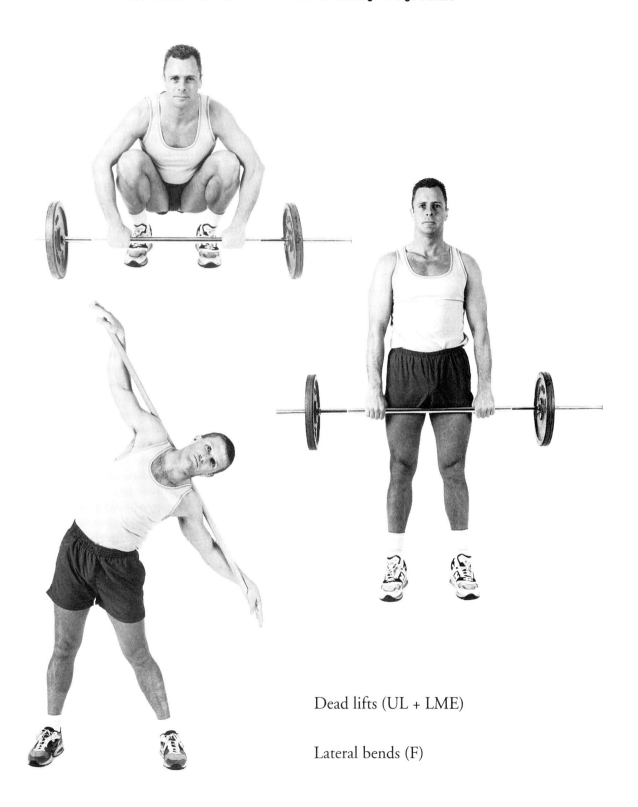

Dead lifts (UL + LME)

Lateral bends (F)

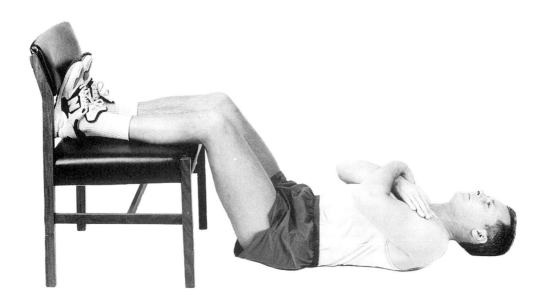

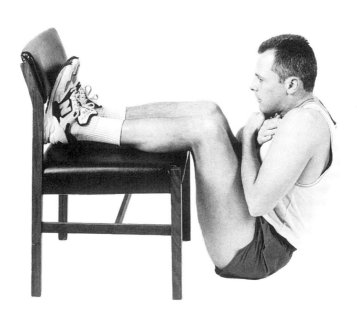

Sit-ups with a chair (A + F + LME) or use an incline bench at the gym.

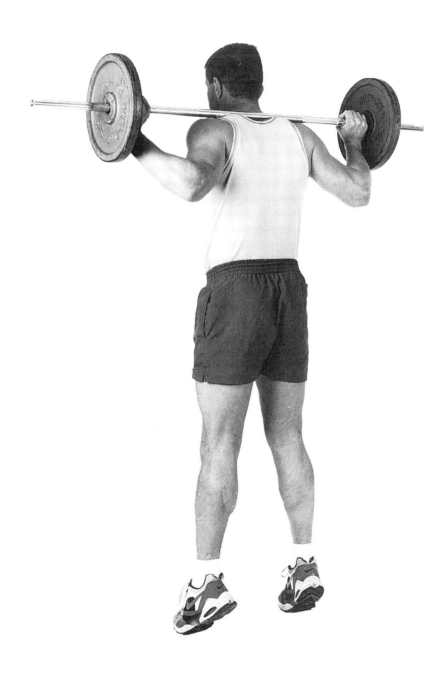

Calf-raising with weights

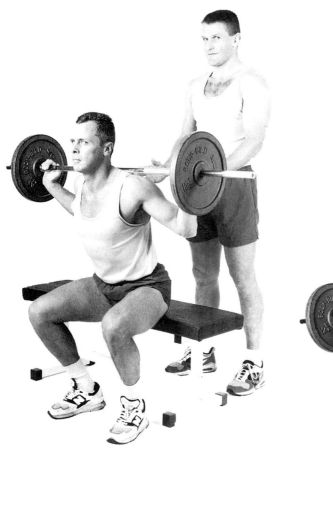

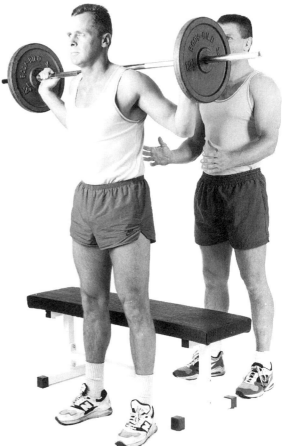

Stand-ups with weights (LME)

Week 13

SESSION 1 (3 HOURS 15 MINS) (B&B)

12-mile (19.2kms) run (+ 35lbs + 9lbs weapon)

Across rough terrain in 2 hours 35 mins.

SESSION 2 (1 HOUR 30 MINS)

Circuit Training

5 sets of 20 reps.

See Week 1, Session 2.

SESSION 3

(3 HOURS 30 MINS) (B&B)

14-mile (22.4kms) run (+ 35lbs + 9lbs weapon)

In 3 hours 2 mins.

SESSION 4 (1 HOUR 30 MINS)

Interval training (see definition at end of chapter.)

See Week 3, Session 1.

- 6 x 400m;
- 8 x 200m;
- 10 x 100m sprints with 100m jog rests.

SESSION 5

(4 HOURS 30 MINS) (B&B)

16-mile (25.6kms) cross country run (+ 30lbs + 9lbs weapon)

In 4 hours.

Week 14

SESSION 1 (1 HOUR 30 MINS)

Swimming

- Jump in.
- Tread water for 2 mins.
- Swim 100m any stroke, no time limit (not allowed to touch sides or bottom of pool).
- Total of 1 hour exercising in pool. (No back stroke. Use variations of arms only, legs only, with floats or pull buoys. Experiment with fartlek in the pool i.e. swim easy for 20m then maximum effort for 20m, climb out and repeat.)
- Climb out at deep end without using steps.

SESSION 2 (1 HOUR 20 MINS)

6-mile fartlek run

In 50 mins. (See definition at end of chapter.)

SESSION 3 (1 HOUR 30 MINS)

Aerobic conditioning and weight training

See Week 12, Session 4.

SESSION 4 (1 HOUR 40 MINS) (B&B)

6.25-mile (10kms) run (+ 30lbs + 9lbs weapon)

To be completed in 68 mins.

SESSION 5 (2 HOURS 10 MINS)

8-mile run (+ 35lbs + 9lbs weapon)

To be completed in 1 hour 36 mins.

Week 15

SESSION 1 (5 HOURS) (B&B)

18-mile (28.8kms) run (+ 35lbs + 9lbs weapon)

To be completed in 4 hours 30 mins.

SESSION 2 (1 HOUR 30 MINS)

Swimming

- Jump in.
- Tread water for 2 mins.
- Swim 100m any stroke, no time limit (not allowed to touch sides or bottom of pool).
- Total of 1 hour exercising in pool (see Week 14, Session 1).
- Climb out at deep end without using steps.

SESSION 3 (1 HOUR 30 MINS)

Gym session

5 sets of 20 reps.

See Week 1, Session 2.

SESSION 4

(1 HOUR 35 MINS) (B&B)

5-mile run with hill reps (+ 35lbs + 9lbs weapon)

At 13 mins/mile pace. See Week 5, Session 4.

SESSION 5

(2 HOURS 20 MINS) (B&B)

10-mile run (+ 35lbs + 9lbs weapon)

In 1 hour 50 mins.

Week 16

SESSION 1 (1 HOUR 20 MINS)

5-mile run

In 50 mins (10 mins/mile pace).

SESSION 2 (1 HOUR 20 MINS)

Aerobic session and weight training

See Week 12, Session 4.

SESSION 3 (2 HOURS) (B&B)

6-mile run (+ 35lbs + 9lbs weapon)

In 1 hour 30 mins.

SESSION 4 (C.1 HOUR) (B&B)

2-mile (3.2kms) run (+ 35lbs + 9lbs weapon)

In under 18 mins.

Congratulations!

You have completed your training. The recruits would now face the daunting prospect of completing P Company Test Week to decide whether they are good enough or not to join The Parachute Regiment. Having completed The Paras Ultimate Fitness you can rest assured that you are an exceptionally fit civilian. No amount of testing can alter that fact. However, if you have a competitive streak and would like to test yourself, the following schedule for one week is a good judge of whether or not you are strong in every area of the training programme.

Test Week

SESSION 1
(2 HOURS 20 MINS) (B&B)

10-mile run (+ 35lbs + 9lbs weapon)

In 1 hour 50 mins.

SESSION 2 (1 HOUR 30 MINS)

Aerobic session and weight training
See Week 12, Session 4.

SESSION 3 (1 HOUR 20 MINS)

6-mile fartlek run

In 50 mins. (See definition at end of chapter.)

SESSION 4 (1 HOUR 30 MINS IN MORNING)

Circuit Training

5 sets of 20 reps.

See Week 1, Session 2.

Followed by afternoon session (1 hour 30 mins)

Swimming

- Jump in.
- Tread water for 2 mins.
- Swim 100m any stroke, no time limit (not allowed to touch sides or bottom of pool).
- Total of 1 hour exercising in pool (see Week 14, Session 1).
- Climb out at deep end without using steps.

SESSION 5
(3 HOURS 30 MINS) (B&B)

14-mile run (+ 35lbs + 9lbs weapon)

In 3 hours 2 mins.

Definition of Running Styles

FARTLEK (MEANING SPEED PLAY) (LL +CR + LME)

This involves running for a set period of time (in our case, 30 mins or more) rather than a specified distance. You vary the pace between flat-out sprints to reasonably fast strides and easy jogging to recover. Choose areas such as woods, bridle paths, parks and sports fields rather than roads for this form of training.

For example, go out for 45–50 mins in the country or a park. Use the first ten mins to warm up, then set your sights on a marker, perhaps a bench, a tree or lamppost, that is half a mile away. Run to that mark, jog until recovered. Pick another mark only 400yds away. Run as fast as you can to get to it and then jog to recover. ('Fast as you can' means exactly that – maximum effort. You will get slower as the session progresses but the effort required should increase. Only you will know if you are giving it all you've got.) You can also run uphill to get your lungs working, or downhill to increase your leg speed. Simply play with bursts of speed and jog to recover.

SPEED REPS (CR + ANAEROBIC)

You need a modern watch with a 'count down' facility or a stopwatch. Set the watch to count down from one minute and set off at a good pace for two minutes. The watch will bleep after 60 seconds so you know when you're half way. At the second bleep, slow to a jog or walk for the next minute. Then repeat. Start by doing 4 of them and then increase this to 6, then to 8, without increasing your speed. When you can do 8 repetitions comfortably, you can start to increase their speed. You would record such a session as: 8 x 2 mins with 1 min jog.

HILL REPS (CR + ANAEROBIC)

This works on strength. Find a suitable hill that is reasonably steep but that you can run up smoothly with controlled effort for 200–400m. Try 6 x 200m repetitions to start with and later build up their length and number. If you settle on 400m attempts, your recovery will be a slow jog back downhill. Start hill training modestly.

INTERVAL TRAINING (CR + ANAEROBIC + TOLERANCE TRAINING TO OVERCOME LOCAL MUSCLE FATIGUE)

This is done on grass or the track. Longer repetitions are a natural progression from a fartlek session. After warm up, start with a two-minute run with speed, followed by a one-minute recovery jog, repeated 6 times:

6 x 2 mins/ 1 min.

Sessions of equivalent intensity but different emphasis can be derived by adjusting any of the numbers involved. Make a distinction between 'full recovery reps' (with a recovery of two minutes or more) and 'partial recovery reps' (with a recovery of one minute). When taking a 'full recovery', opt for longer reps i.e. 3 or 4 mins. You may find the following examples helpful.

FULL RECOVERY REPETITIONS ON GRASS:

- 6–8 x 3 mins/2–3 mins recovery
- 5–6 x 4 mins/2–3 mins recovery
- 4–5 x 5 mins/2–3 mins recovery

(Heart Rate should recover to resting levels i.e. aerobic range of 60–70% of Maximum Heart Rate e.g. MHR of 185 recovers to 130. Repeat.)

PARTIAL RECOVERY REPETITIONS ON TRACK:

- 12 x 400m/100m jog
- 8 x 800m/100m jog
- 5 x (600m/200m jog, 300m/100m jog)

Your Circuit/Gym Training Log				
Exercise	Reps Done	Time Taken	Target Time	Date
Squats:				
Sit-ups:				
Squat Thrusts:				
Dorsal Raises:				
Press-ups:				
Step-ups:				
Twist Sit-ups:				
Leg Lifts:				
Squat Thrusts (Burpees):				
Leg Raises:				
Dips:				
Advanced Dorsal:				

Running Log				
Date	Distance	Time Taken	Target Time	Style e.g. Fartlek + Length/Reps

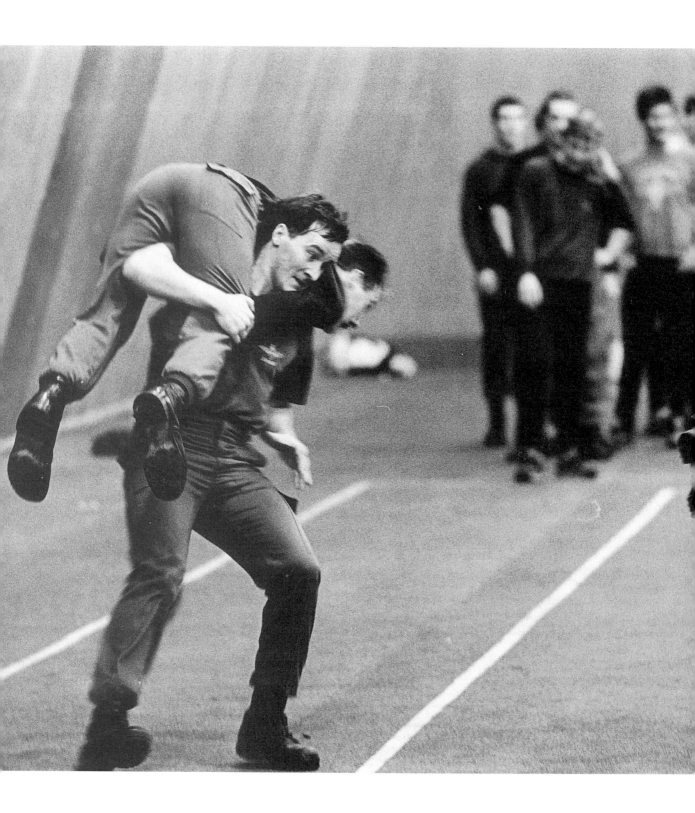

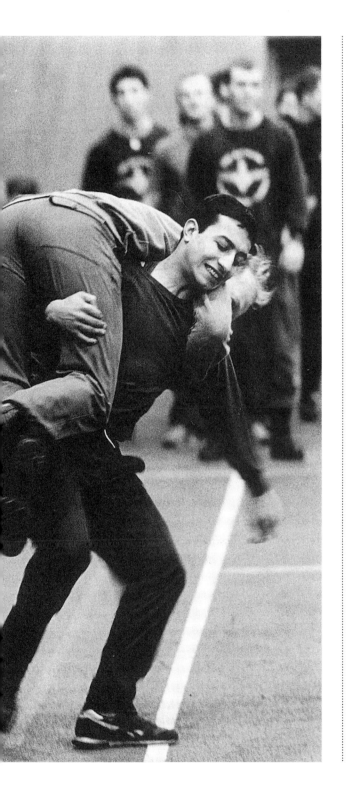

Chapter Eight

Maintaining Fitness

• •

You have done exceptionally well to have achieved this level of fitness. Regrettably, you will not continue to reap its benefits unless you put in some continued effort. The Paras, after all, are effectively full-time athletes with regular fitness sessions, marches and runs built in to Battalion life. They cannot afford to underestimate the physical demands of battle and must be ready at all times to be called away to some hot spot in the world at short notice. In fact, most Paras complement their Battalion training with their own fitness schedule which usually includes running (suckers for punishment, eh?), cycling and recreational sports (if you can call the way they play squash recreational!).

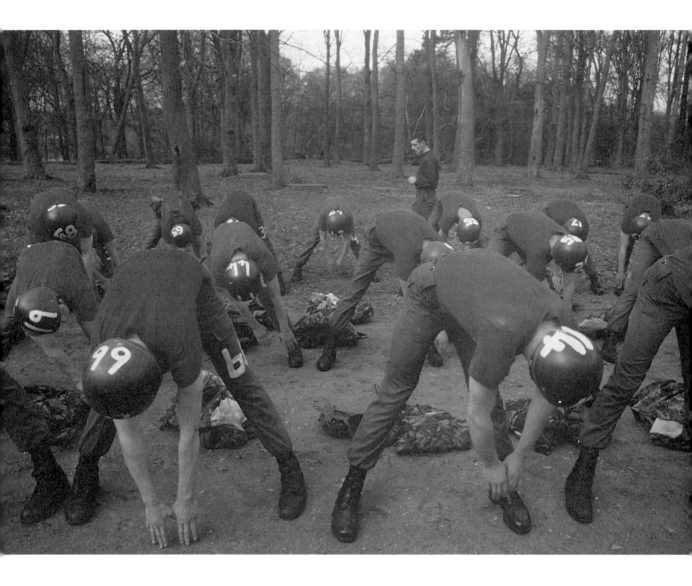

When you have a full-time job and other social and domestic commitments, it is hard to keep up the level of training that you have maintained during the past 16 weeks. The good news is that you can still stay fit by putting in fewer sessions a week. There are those who become hooked on exercise and the adrenalin rush it produces. Even in the Regiment there are those who become addicted to running and train every day, including Christmas Day. In the civilian world, there are aerobics fanatics who attend several classes a day and who feel guilty if they miss one. This is when fitness has become an addiction and, like any obsessive behaviour, it is destructive rather than beneficial. While enjoying your new-found ultimate fitness, you should keep in perspective the fact that you are now an extremely fit civilian but not a full-time athlete. Maintenance is now what you should be aiming for.

Even without training, there is a residual fitness in the body for a short period of time and this disappears more slowly, the fitter you are. In fact, professional athletes can have a break from training of a couple of weeks, and within several days of resuming training, they are back to performance standard. Mere mortals like the rest of us, however, lose our fitness very much more quickly, after a matter of days, in fact.

It is generally accepted that a minimum of three training sessions a week of not less than 20 minutes duration will maintain your fitness level. A better guide is to make sure that during your training periods, your heart rate is raised to 60–85% of its maximum rate for at least 20 minutes. In effect, allowing time for warm-up and cool-down, you are looking at a minimum of a 45-minute training session, three times a week.

What To Do

Throughout The Paras Ultimate Fitness Training Programme, you will have discovered elements that you enjoy, those you could do without and some you positively detest. The likelihood of you continuing to train is increased if you are doing something that you enjoy. So, look at those aspects of the training and incorporate them into your maintenance programme. Since the goal is always overall body conditioning, you must now identify those areas of fitness which are being neglected – for example, if you are concentrating on running, the aerobic element of your programme is nicely taken care of but, unless you are running with weight, the strength element and flexibility are missing. In this case, circuit or weight training plus stretching or plyometrics would be an ideal complement to your running sessions. There are numerous activities from which to choose and recreational or competitive sports can be used as variations so that your fitness maintenance does not become monotonous. A rough comparison of activities and their physiological benefits can be found later in this chapter.

Remember to follow the golden rules of training that applied during the 16-week programme. Although you are not training to the same intense degree, there is still a need to warm up properly, concentrating on stretching well, keeping the heart beating strongly for at least 20 and preferably 30 minutes, before a gradual warm-down. Don't be tempted to cut corners simply because you've reached your goal. Injuries such as pulled muscles can still happen even in recreational activities. Fit your three to 5 training sessions into a 7 day week making sure you break up the sessions with proper rest days i.e. don't cram them all into the weekend. A weekly maintenance programme may look something like this:

- Sunday: Long-distance run.
- Monday: Rest.
- Tuesday: Swimming.
- Wednesday: Circuit Training.
- Thursday: Rest.
- Friday: Plyometrics.
- Saturday: Golf.

Finally, enjoy being fit. You can accommodate your training into a normal lifestyle and still enjoy socializing and letting your hair down. There is nothing worse than a fitness bore who is 'holier than thou' at a party. Paras are renowned for partying as hard as they train. Have fun – you've got the energy to do it now and still feel great the next day!

Sporting Comparisons

There is no direct equivalent for different exercises since there are so many variables in the standard of skill, the intensity of play, the terrain, etc. So the suggested alternatives below are only a rough guide. As a basic rule of thumb, if you exercise hard and get your heart rate up, all these activities will have much the same beneficial effects within their area of influence, that is to say aerobic, strength or overall conditioning.

Aerobic Alternatives

- Running.
- Cycling.
- Swimming.
- Racket sports:
  badminton (45 mins minimum);

squash (45 mins minimum);

tennis (one hour minimum).

- Ball sports:

soccer (60–90 mins minimum,
but 5-a-side is even better);

rugby (a full game but 7-a-side is
better still);

basketball (30 mins minimum);

volleyball (full game);

hockey (full game).

Strength Alternatives

- Rowing (either on the river or a machine).
- Golf (play 18 holes at a rapid pace and carry your own bag).
- Weight training (one hour minimum under supervision).
- Horse riding (one hour minimum, but not to be undertaken if you are a novice).
- Windsurfing (45 mins minimum but again, not for beginners).

- Circuit training (45 mins minimum).

Combining Strength and Aerobic Activity

- High impact/low impact/step aerobics (45-minute work-out minimum).
- Skiing (full day).
- Waterpolo (full game).
- Dancing (one hour minimum).

Although you are simply maintaining your levels of fitness, play to the best of your ability whether you are playing a competitive or recreational sport, and that way you will virtually guarantee that you are getting the optimum fitness effects. By that, I do not mean winning at all costs. In fact, it is a good idea to play with people who are of a better standard than yourself as this tends to raise your game and stretch you a little more.

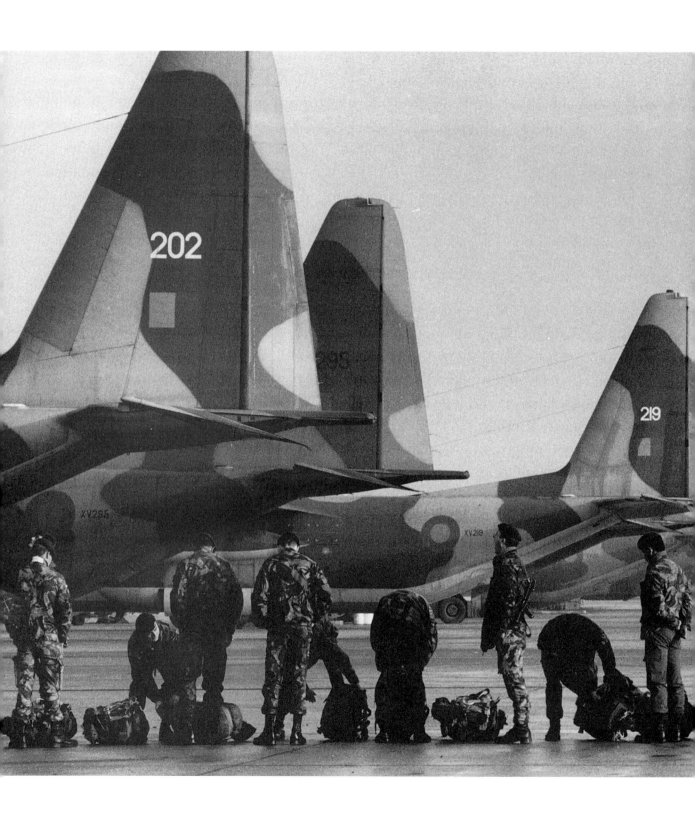

Chapter Nine

Conclusion

• •

I have no idea what motivated you to get fit in the first place, nor what prompted you to choose this particular programme. However, if you have completed the 16-week course, I know that I can respect you – your determination, strength of character and sheer guts are unquestionable.

I also know that you are now an exceptionally fit individual and that you will be enjoying not only the obvious benefits of a well-conditioned body but also the heightened sense of self-esteem that overcoming a challenge such as this brings. I suspect too that you will be determined to maintain your fitness; you will not readily return to your previous fitness levels; and you will always eschew a 'couch potato' lifestyle.

With enough strength of character to see yourself through such an arduous programme, you don't need me to tell you that you have really achieved something special. Yet, allow me to say a hearty 'Well Done' and to encourage you to keep up the good work. You have proved to us all that you really are Utrinque Paratus – Ready for Anything.

Fancy jumping out of a plane next?